WORKING WITH ADOLESCENT VIOLENCE AND ABUSE TOWARDS PARENTS

Adolescent violence and abuse towards parents is increasingly recognised as a global problem. Inverting how we normally understand power to operate in abusive relationships, it involves actors who cannot easily be categorised as victims or perpetrators, and often impacts families who are facing multiple stressors and hardships and may be experiencing other forms of family abuse. This unique book draws on an international selection of contributors to identify, present and explore what we know about what works when supporting these families.

Exploring conceptual and theoretical challenges produced by this emerging social problem:

- Part 1 discusses some well-established intervention approaches and programmes, looking at their theoretical base and relevant assessment, delivery and evaluation issues. It provides readers with a theoretical framework and toolkit for use in their own intervention work.
- Part 2 presents examples of innovative practice, with an emphasis on diverse institutional settings, geographical locations and other important contexts that shape practice. It provides readers with an understanding of some of the complexities involved in this kind of intervention work, offering tools and strategies to be applied in their own work.

This interdisciplinary guide provides an essential resource for students and practitioners with an interest in domestic and family violence, youth studies, child protection, drug and alcohol work, and youth justice from a wide range of professional backgrounds.

Amanda Holt, PhD, is Reader in Criminology at the University of Roehampton, London, UK. She works from an interdisciplinary perspective, drawing on ideas from psychology, sociology, social policy and social work. Her research interests primarily focus on families, identity and harm, and she has published widely on the topic of adolescent violence and abuse towards parents, including the book *Adolescent-to-Parent Abuse: Current Understandings in Research, Policy and Practice* (2013). She has also published empirical and theoretical research on a number of other criminological topics, including anti-violence strategies in schools, parenting and youth justice, and qualitative methodologies.

WORKING WITH ADOLESCENT VIOLENCE AND ABUSE TOWARDS PARENTS

Approaches and contexts for intervention

Edited by
Amanda Holt

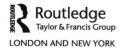

Routledge
Taylor & Francis Group

LONDON AND NEW YORK

First published 2016
by Routledge
2 Park Square, Milton Park, Abingdon, Oxon OX14 4RN

and by Routledge
711 Third Avenue, New York, NY 10017

Routledge is an imprint of the Taylor & Francis Group, an information business

British Library Cataloguing-in-Publication Data
A catalogue record for this book is available from the British Library

Library of Congress Cataloging in Publication Data
Working with adolescent violence and abuse towards parents: approaches and contexts for intervention/edited by Amanda Holt.
  p.; cm.
  Includes bibliographical references and index.
  I. Holt, Amanda, editor.
  [DNLM: 1. Adolescent. 2. Social Behavior Disorders. 3. Domestic Violence. 4. Parent–Child Relations. 5. Psychology, Adolescent. WS 463]
  RJ506.V56
  616.85′8200835 – dc23
  2015007312

ISBN: 978-1-138-80799-0 (hbk)
ISBN: 978-1-138-80801-0 (pbk)
ISBN: 978-1-315-75078-1 (ebk)

Typeset in Bembo and Stone Sans
by Florence Production Ltd, Stoodleigh, Devon, UK

CONTENTS

ILLUSTRATIONS

CONTRIBUTORS

Lily Anderson, MSW, has been working with the Step-Up program since 1997. Lily co-developed Step-Up and co-authored the Step-Up curriculum. She has worked in the field of domestic violence since 1978, including work with survivors, perpetrators and parents. Lily developed and authored a parenting curriculum for the Family Services Domestic Violence Treatment Program in Seattle and coordinated the program from 1986 to 1998. In 1997, she co-authored a curriculum for parents of children who have experienced domestic violence, *Helping Children who have Experienced Domestic Violence: A Guide for Parents*, which is used nationwide in perpetrator and survivor programmes.

Fiona Barakat BSc, MSc, PGCE is a lecturer at Westminster Kingsway College in London, UK. Fiona is trained in counselling psychology and for the past 11 years has worked at DVIP in London, supporting women who have experienced domestic violence. She was also part of developing and delivering the Yuva project and delivers workshops and training on domestic violence and its impacts on families, young people and children, and on working with domestic violence within a cultural context, having worked bilingually with both Arabic- and English-speaking clients.

Kristin Whitehill Bolton, PhD, MSW, is Assistant Professor at the School of Social Work, University of North Carolina, USA. She has published peer-reviewed articles, presented at both national and international conferences, and serves on the Solution Focused Brief Therapy Association Research Committee. In 2012, she was the recipient of a research grant from the SFBTA to conduct a programme evaluation on youth violent offenders in Tarrant County, Texas.

Kathleen Daly, PhD, is Professor of Criminology and Criminal Justice at Griffith University (Brisbane, Australia). She writes on gender, race, crime and justice, and has produced numerous books, journal articles and law reviews. In the past decade, she has conducted research on restorative justice, contemporary forms of Indigenous justice and transitional justice, with a focus on innovative justice practices for domestic, sexual and family violence. Her book, *Redressing Institutional Abuse of Children* (2014, Palgrave Macmillan), examines the emergence of the social problem of institutional abuse of children and the redress mechanisms used in 19 major Canadian and Australian cases of historical abuse.

Jane Evans is a parenting specialist, Global Academy expert, freelance trainer and writer. She has over 20 years' experience working with children and families affected by domestic abuse, adolescent-to-parent abuse, mental illness, substance dependency and other complex needs. Jane regularly appears on television and radio to discuss matters relating to children and parenting, and is a regular expert contributor to *Social Work Helper, UK Fostering* and *Adoption UK* magazines. Jane's work with young children and parents affected by living with domestic violence has informed her acclaimed story book series, *How are You Feeling Today Baby Bear?* (2014, Jessica Kingsley).

Eddie Gallagher is a psychologist, social worker, family therapist and trainer who has been working with families and youth for 40 years in a range of settings (in the UK and Australia). He currently has a private practice in Melbourne, Australia. He has a long-term interest in family violence generally and runs men's behaviour change groups. For over 20 years he has had a focus on violence towards parents, working with over 400 families where this has occurred. He developed the Who's in Charge? group programme for parents abused by their children.

Amanda Holt, PhD, is Reader in Criminology at the University of Roehampton, London. She works from an interdisciplinary perspective, drawing on ideas from psychology, sociology, social policy and social work. Her research interests primarily focus on families, identity and harm, and she has published widely on the topic of adolescent violence and abuse towards parents, including the book *Adolescent-to-Parent Abuse: Current Understandings in Research, Policy and Practice* (Policy Press, 2013). She has also published empirical and theoretical research on a number of other criminological topics, including anti-violence strategies in schools, parenting and youth justice, and qualitative methodologies.

Jo Howard is a social worker and family therapist based in Melbourne, Australia. She has published extensively, including *Mothers and Sons: Bringing Up Boys as a Sole Parent* and a parenting manual, *Bringing Up Boys*. Her 15-year contribution to adolescent family violence includes playing a key role in the development of government-funded programmes, inclusion of the issue of adolescent family violence into family violence policy and research. In 2009 she gained a Winston Churchill Fellowship to research best practice responses to adolescent family violence across the United States and Canada. She delivers training to a broad range of sectors in working with adolescent family violence and supports implementation of concurrent parent/adolescent programmes across Australia.

Catheleen Jordan, PhD, is Professor and holder of the Cheryl Milkes Moore Professorship in Mental Health at the University of Texas at Arlington, School of Social Work. Catheleen is an internationally known scholar and leader in family social work assessment and intervention. In addition to her scholarly publications, she is the author of several books, including *An Introduction to Family Social Work* (with Collins and Coleman) and *Clinical Assessment for Social Workers* (with Franklin). She was recently awarded the Texas state lifetime achievement award from NASW where she was Texas State President from 2007 to 2009.

Gjori Langeland has worked in the domestic violence field for 15 years. She is a senior manager at DVIP and a Trustee of Desta, a voluntary sector consortium working within health and social care. Her involvement in developing services for adult perpetrators and victims, and for children and young people affected by domestic abuse at DVIP, includes the pilot of a domestic abuse and parenting service focusing on parenting in the aftermath of domestic abuse and the inception and ongoing development of the Yuva service.

Peter Lehmann, PhD, LCSW, is Associate Professor of Social Work at the University of Texas at Arlington, TX. His research focus is on assessing and developing strategies of change with youth and adult offender populations that focus on competency and strengths, and which are partnership based.

Ester McGeeney, PhD, is a youth researcher and practitioner with over 10 years' experience working with young people and families in a range of different settings. Ester has previously worked for DVIP and was involved in developing and delivering the Yuva service. She currently works for the UK sexual health charity Brook where she has recently completed *The 'Good Sex' Project: Building Evidence Based Practice in Young People's Sexual Health*. Ester's research is principally in the fields of youth, gender and sexuality. She has a particular interest in creative and participatory methods of research and knowledge exchange.

Latesha Murphy-Edwards, PhD, is a registered clinical psychologist with over 17 years' experience working within community mental health and hospital settings. She currently holds a part-time position at the Southern District Health Board's Child, Adolescent and Family Service (Invercargill, New Zealand). Latesha also prepares specialist psychology reports for the Youth Court. Her doctorate research at the University of Canterbury, New Zealand was on the topic of adolescent-to-parent domestic property violence.

Haim Omer, PhD, is Professor of Clinical Psychology at Tel Aviv University and founder of the Parent Training Clinic at Schneider Children's Medical Center of Israel. He has written many books and papers on the psychology of children, including the influential *Non-Violent Resistance: A New Approach to Violent and Self-Destructive Children* (2004). He developed the 'non-violent resistance' approach to parent training, which is now used by practitioners working with parents across the developed world.

Roberto Pereira is a psychiatrist, Senior Consultant and Head of Unit of Mental Health in the Basque Health Service in Spain. He is also accredited by the Spanish Federation of Psychotherapy as a couples' and family psychotherapist, teacher and supervisor, and is currently Vice President of the Spanish and Latin American Network of Systemic Schools. He is Director of the Vasco-Navarra School of Family Therapy and also Director of the Euskarri Intervention Center for Filio-Parental Violence. He has authored numerous papers and texts on filio-parental violence, and provides training courses in Europe and Latin America on this subject.

Gregory Routt has an MA in Counseling Psychology from Antioch University in Seattle, United States, and has been working with the Step-Up program since it began in 1997. Greg co-developed the programme and co-authored the Step-Up curriculum. Prior to Step-Up, he worked with adult perpetrators of domestic violence at Family Services Domestic Violence Treatment Program in Seattle and was co-director of the programme. Greg has also worked as a substance abuse counsellor with inmates in the King County Jail, Seattle, USA.

Dannielle Wade is a Research Assistant in the Key Centre for Ethics, Law, Justice, and Governance, Griffith University (Brisbane, Australia). She works with Professor Kathleen Daly on innovative justice research projects. She has a BA of Laws (Hons) and Criminology and Criminal Justice from Griffith University. Dannielle is a volunteer for the Griffith University Innocence Project, which aims to exonerate factually innocent people wrongfully convicted in Australia.

Shem Williams has worked in the domestic violence field for around seven years, in the UK and Australia. In this field he has worked with adult perpetrators and victims of domestic violence, young people who use violence and abuse in their close relationships (including towards family members) and training professionals in how to respond effectively to domestic and child-to-parent violence. Shem was closely involved in the development and delivery of DVIP's Yuva young people's service, which works with young people who are using abuse in close relationships and their partners/family members.

FOREWORD

Barbara Cottrell

For way too long, parent abuse has been a hidden form of family violence. The result has been that many families have not received the help they need. Often this was because people did not know how to help. *Working with Adolescent Violence and Abuse towards Parents: Approaches and Contexts for Intervention* will contribute to changing that. It was nearly 20 years ago when a family counselor told me that two of her clients were being beaten by their teenage children. She was at her wits' end because no one seemed to know anything about this form of family violence. To help her, I started researching the topic. She was right: there was little information available. Most people had never heard of such a thing. Most people, that is, except for service providers. When I asked social workers, police and even teachers if they had ever encountered parent abuse in their work, many said they had but I was the first person who had asked about it. And they had no idea how to help.

We now know much more about parent abuse. We know these parents are usually in a state of despair and desperately need help. In spite of the crippling shame they suffer, some do turn to family and friends or to service providers. But all too often no help is available. However, thanks to scholars like Amanda Holt, that is changing. Dr. Holt has brought together service providers from around the world who have decades of experience working with these families. Here they detail the ways they give support. They offer their insights. For the first time, in one document, we can read about parent abuse in North America, Europe, Australia, New Zealand and Asia. From this book we can learn about programs that are successfully supporting families to end the abuse.

Using real case studies, the authors describe their assessment, delivery and evaluation methods in a wide variety of programs, some well established, others newer initiatives. It is fascinating to read how they deal with some of the contradictions and challenges they face. The similarities in places as different as the

United States, Australia, Spain, England and Israel are also intriguing. We can learn from them all. One of the book's authors, Jane Evans, captures how I feel when she states, "It is encouraging that there is now a global 'curiosity' about this issue because the more 'parent abuse' is talked and written about, the more parents may feel they can reach out for the support they need and deserve." We can learn a lot about how to support families from this book, which shows there are places all over the world where services are being offered, and families successfully helped.

Barbara Cottrell
Adjunct Professor
St Mary's University, Halifax, Nova Scotia, Canada

ACKNOWLEDGEMENTS

This book would not have been possible without the enthusiasm and support of all of the contributors, and I thank them all for their insightful and articulate chapters. The work they do is inspiring, and their wide-ranging knowledge and experience in this field have given this book authenticity and credibility. Our shared hope is that this volume makes an important contribution to current debates about how we might work with this most complex of problems to help eliminate violence and abuse from families' lives. I would also like to thank Jenny Bright, Barbara Cottrell, Jo Howard and Sam Lewis, who have been so generous with their support and feedback during the development of this collection.

INTRODUCTION

Working with adolescent violence and abuse towards parents

Amanda Holt

This book is about a very particular problem. It involves a pattern of behaviour, instigated by a child or young person, which involves using verbal, financial, physical and/or emotional means to practise power and exert control over a parent. The power that is practised is, to some extent, *intentional*, and the *control* that is exerted over a parent is achieved through fear, such that a parent unhealthily adapts his/her own behaviour to accommodate the child. Commonly reported abusive behaviours include name-calling, threats to harm self or others, attempts at humiliation, damage to property, theft and physical violence. Like other forms of family violence, it can produce devastating short-term and long-term harms to those who are subject to it. These harms include emotional distress (including worry, grief and despair); physical and mental health problems (including anxiety, depression and suicide ideation); problems in personal, family and social relationships; and knock-on effects on work and finances (Cottrell, 2004; Holt, 2013). Furthermore, the abuse and violence can impact upon all family members, including the adolescent him-herself, who may experience increasing isolation and be involved in other offending behaviour (Laurent and Derry, 1999), including later violence targeted towards dating partners (LaPorte *et al.*, 2009) and marriage partners (O'Leary *et al.*, 2004).

While many practitioners have documented an apparent increase in the visibility of this problem, it is important to recognise that this is not a 'new' phenomenon – historical records going back as far as the seventeenth century have documented young people's violence towards parents and evidence suggests that such violence was taken more seriously, and dealt with more punitively, than any other form of violence (Miettinen, 2014). It is also not a 'Western' problem that can be easily explained away in terms of cultural shifts in parenting practices – its incidence has been reported in Taiwan (Hsu *et al.*, 2014), South Korea (Kim *et al.*, 2008), Egypt (Fawzi *et al.*, 2013), Sri Lanka (Perera, 2006) and Colombia (Betancourt, 2012).

What is new is that, over the past twenty years or so, a number of practitioners have identified adolescent violence and abuse towards parents as a problem that needs to be taken seriously and that requires specialised ways of working. Existing agencies that respond to families in need (such as the police, child protection agencies, schools, health services) often struggle to respond to this complex problem within the confines of their resources and policy frameworks. As such, it is difficult to see where parents can go for help. Should parents call the police following an incident of violence from their son or daughter? Research suggests that often police do not take this form of family violence seriously and blame the parent for their child's behaviour. In any case, parents are understandably reluctant to set in place a chain of events that may lead to the criminalisation of their child. Should parents call child protection services? Such responses are often met with a refusal to take the case on because the child in question does not meet the (very high) threshold of harm required for such statutory involvement. Should parents call domestic violence support agencies? This might be useful in terms of providing emotional support and developing safety plans, but particular support strategies that are set up to respond to violence between adults are often inappropriate when applied to children (to whom parents have a legal responsibility). Should parents call mental health services? This may be useful if a child is experiencing mental health problems, but what if – as in many cases – the child is not? So what can be done to help parents and families who are struggling with this most complex of problems? This book, written by practitioners and researchers who work across a number of sectors, aims to provide answers to this question. And as the following section highlights, this question is a pressing one.

What do we know about adolescent violence and abuse towards parents?

It is always difficult to research family violence because great efforts tend to be made by family members to hide the problem. Furthermore, abuse is often not recognised as such within families – it can become so normalised that it is 'just the way things are'. Therefore, researchers need to think carefully about how they can sensitively ask the right questions that will lead to disclosure about experiences of abuse and violence. However, as in all social research, the way questions are asked tends to shape the answers that are given. For example, research on this topic often suggests that adolescent abuse towards parents affects 5–15 per cent of all families. This statistic is based on community surveys (i.e. those that ask a sample from the general population) and tend to focus on the *frequency* of *physical abuse* (e.g. how often have you hit your parent? Or, how often has your child hit you, in the last 12 months?). Large datasets are subject to statistical analysis and prevalence rates are produced (e.g. see Peek *et al.*, 1985; Agnew and Huguley, 1989; Ullman and Straus, 2003). However, such methods fail to produce the contextual information that might tell us whether such data actually fit into our definition in terms of a *pattern* of behaviour that produces *harmful outcomes*.[1]

Rather than asking questions of large populations, some researchers ask questions of criminal justice data. For example, what are the numbers and characteristics of young people arrested, charged or convicted of an offence against a parent? (e.g. Condry and Miles, 2014; Contreras and Cano, 2014; Purcell *et al.*, 2014). This method is more likely to capture those extreme cases where families have reached crisis point amid ongoing patterns of abusive behaviour and the police have intervened. Similarly, practitioners can ask questions of family members who have come forward and sought support for their experiences of abuse and violence from their children. Through observations and interviews, this method can produce rich and insightful data about the dynamics of this problem and how it can be managed, as well as the kinds of families who seek support from different kinds of practitioners. However, neither criminal justice data nor service-user data can offer 'prevalence rates' since we do not know what the 'dark figure' is – that is, the number of families who are suffering in silence. The brief summary of research findings that follows, which draws on community survey data, criminal justice data and service-user data, needs to be interpreted in terms of these methodological limitations.

Adolescent abuse and violence and the families who experience it

Like all forms of family violence, we know that adolescent abuse and violence towards parents is highly gendered. Whichever method of data collection is used, mothers are found to be the most victimised, and this pattern is particularly pronounced when examining criminal justice and service-user data, where the ratio is as high as 8:2 (see Condry and Miles, 2014; O'Connor, 2007; Perera, 2006). There are various reasons for this, related to the way most families are configured (e.g. mothers spend more time with their children) and how women are constructed as the 'ideal victim' of abuse and violence (see Christie, 1986). It would also appear that most of the abuse and violence is instigated by sons, rather than daughters. Again, the difference is particularly pronounced within criminal justice and service-user data where the more 'entrenched' cases are likely to be found (e.g. O'Connor, 2007; Strom *et al.*, 2014; Purcell *et al.*, 2014). While those social and cultural reasons that may explain female victimisation may also explain the disproportion of sons' instigation of abuse, such explanations are not sufficient: daughters do instigate abuse and fathers are also victimised (see Daly and Wade, this volume). It is also important to recognise that siblings are also often victimised – both directly, and indirectly through the impact of living in an abusive household – and research has so far found little evidence of gendered violence in this context.

In terms of social class, socio-demographic status and ethnicity, there is currently little robust evidence to support any particular pattern. Very often, reports that suggest a preponderance of particular social class populations in particular research settings (e.g. see Charles, 1986) can be explained in terms of the kind of support that particular groups will seek out i.e. those that have money may seek support from a private therapist, while those without such resources may be limited to seeking support from statutory agencies. However, such patterns are complex. We know that a disproportionate number of parents who come into contact with professionals because of adolescent abuse and violence are from single-parent households (Condry and Miles, 2014; Contreras and Cano, 2014). We also know from sociological research that single-parent households tend to be headed by women and they are also likely to experience a disproportionate amount of poverty (see Pearce, 1978) and that domestic violence more generally is linked with poverty and stress (Goodman et al., 2009). Untangling these complexities within the context of adolescent abuse and violence towards parents is a continuing research challenge.

In terms of age, most research in this field has restricted its age parameters to the teenage years (i.e. ages 13–19). The peak age of young people's involvement in the criminal justice system because of related offences is around 15 years (Nowakowski and Mattern, 2014; Strom et al., 2014). However, parents often report that the abusive behaviour from their child started earlier than this, sometimes from as young as 5 years of age. In other cases, parents report that abusive behaviour appeared more suddenly, often at the onset of adolescence (i.e. around 12 years). Thus, as is the case more generally in terms of adolescent offending, it is possible that there are at least two age-related pathways into adolescent abuse and violence towards parents. Applying Moffit's (1993) taxonomy, there may be the more common 'adolescence-limited' abusive behaviour, which emerges during the teenage years and then decreases over time, and a rarer 'life-course persistent' abuse, which begins much earlier and persists into adulthood. Aside from Shon and Barton-Bellessa's (2012) work on parricide (that is, *fatal* violence towards parents), little research has examined this problem from this developmental perspective. However, some developmental insights can be gained by exploring the different contexts in which adolescent abuse and violence towards parents takes place.

Pathways to adolescent-to-parent abuse

Research that has looked at the contexts in which adolescent abuse and violence takes place can be informative in identifying hypotheses as to why it happens. However, as many of the contributors to this volume point out, there is unlikely to be any single explanation for any individual case. Research has explored a number of potential pathways that will be briefly discussed here: neurodevelopmental disorders; mental health and/or substance misuse problems; previous family violence and parenting practices.

Sometimes, *neurodevelopmental disorders*[2] such as autism spectrum disorder (ASD) and attention deficit hyperactivity disorder (ADHD) may be implicated in aggressive behaviour towards parents. Some studies have examined the prevalence of such diagnoses within clinical populations where there is child-to-parent aggression and have identified above-average numbers of children with a neurodevelopmental diagnosis in such populations (e.g. see Laurent and Derry, 1999; Perera, 2006; González-Álvarez et al., 2010). Other studies have focused on a single disorder (e.g. ADHD) and looked at it in terms of the proportion of cases that feature child aggression towards parents (e.g. Ghanizadeh and Jafari, 2010). It is often difficult to compare these studies because of cultural differences in diagnosis, changing clinical definitions of diagnostic categories, and because the samples are taken from psychiatric populations where inevitably there will be above-average prevalence rates for psychiatric disorders. At a conceptual level it is questionable whether such cases should come within the definition of 'abuse' or 'violence' at all because issues of *control* and *intentionality* are so much more complicated – indeed, some researchers specifically exclude such cases from their definition (e.g. see Aroca Montolio *et al.*, 2013). However, aggression towards parents from children is not an inevitable symptom of any particular neurodevelopmental disorder. Thus, while it might present a particular *pathway* to such challenging behaviour, it is not its *cause*, and – as this book will testify – much can be done to help parents find ways of managing their child's aggression within such contexts.

Mental health problems in young people are frequently reported by practitioners who work with adolescent abuse and violence towards parents, and this appears to be consistent across different types of research samples and across different countries (e.g. Kennedy *et al.*, 2010; Routt and Anderson, 2011; Ibabe *et al.*, 2014). Problems most frequently reported include post-traumatic stress disorder (PTSD), depression, anxiety problems and suicide ideation and/or suicide attempts. Relatedly, *substance misuse* problems have been found to be implicated in many cases of abusive behaviour towards parents (e.g. Pagani *et al.*, 2004, 2009; Pelletier and Coutu, 1992). However, this link appears to be indirect, in that an adolescent's use of substances produces more conflict in the parent–child relationship, rather than because the young person is 'under the influence' during abusive interactions (although of course this may happen).

Family violence pathways are also common. Some surveys have identified links between abuse towards parents and parental aggression towards children (e.g. Brezina, 1999; Margolin and Baucom, 2014). Other studies have identified histories of intimate partner violence (IPV) in families where there is current adolescent abuse towards parents (Ullman and Straus, 2003; Boxer *et al.*, 2009). There are a number of explanations for these patterns, including learning and imitating behaviour from the abusive parent; the impact of trauma that growing up in such households can produce; and – in cases where the parents are now separated – anger towards the resident parent (usually the mother) for instigating the parental separation. Certainly, research that has gathered accounts from mothers who are experiencing abuse from their children has found that many mothers frame their child's abusive behaviour towards them within these explanatory frameworks (see Holt, 2013: 73–74).

Finally, links between *parenting practices* and adolescent abuse towards parents have been researched, perhaps more extensively than any other pathway. Particular interest in such correlations may, to some extent, be explained by the dominance of *parental determinism* – an explanatory framework that is frequently invoked to explain all problematic teenage behaviour in terms of poor parenting practices.[3]

Research has identified links between adolescent abuse towards parents and 'permissive parenting', 'inconsistent parenting' and a lack of positive reinforcement from parents (Paulson et al., 1990; Peek et al., 1985; Jablonski, 2007). Quality of attachment bond between parent and child has also been examined, with surveys finding links between abusive behaviour towards parents and young people *not feeling close to parents, not feeling emotionally rewarded by parents* and *not feeling in agreement with their parents* (Agnew and Huguley, 1989; Paulson et al., 1990; Peek et al., 1985). However, such correlational research studies need to be interpreted appropriately, because it is likely that any such correlations are *bi-directional*, in that parental experiences of abuse from their child will in turn shape their own parenting practices and the quality of emotional bond they have with their child. Furthermore, other factors will also play a role both in the adolescent's abusive behaviour and in parenting practices (such as a mother's experience of partner abuse in the family home).

The summary of research presented here is not to suggest that there are no other pathways into abusive behaviour towards parents, or indeed that there are always clear pathways – in some cases, no 'obvious' routes can be identified (Condry and Miles, 2014; Vink et al., 2014). And cases where there is no particular pathway raise complicated questions as to how any intervention work should proceed.

Experiencing adolescent violence and abuse towards parents

Qualitative studies that have explored parents' experiences of abuse and violence from their child have identified common patterns in the emergence of the abusive dynamic (e.g. Cottrell, 2004; Jackson, 2003; Eckstein, 2004; Haw, 2010). It tends to start gradually, beginning with verbal abuse before escalating into forms of physical abuse and/or emotional abuse. This perceived behavioural trajectory operates alongside a parent's emotional trajectory, which often begins with disbelief and denial and develops into fear and worry, self-blame and shame, resentment and betrayal and, ultimately, hopelessness and despair. Such emotions are understandable given the hidden nature of the abuse, the parent-blame culture that shapes common responses to 'difficult' adolescent behaviour and the biological, emotional and legal bonds that are written into the child–parent relationship. Yet while such emotions are understandable, support for such families is frequently patchy and often non-existent. Practitioners and researchers who have recognised the need to respond to the problem have often had to operate in a landscape where there is little (if any) policy guidance and few (if any) resources. Whether working in healthcare, youth justice, domestic violence, counselling and/or research settings, it is to their credit that they have developed unique ways of working with families where an adolescent is behaving abusively and/or violently towards their parent(s). I feel privileged that many of these pioneering practitioners and researchers have contributed chapters to this unique volume.

A word about words

While many of the contributors to this volume identify the importance of *naming the problem*, there is no consensus on what to call it. In some ways, it is desirable that there is consistency in terminology – it has implications for literature searching and producing a coherent body of knowledge, as well as how we measure its prevalence and conduct comparative research in this field. However, for a problem that is only just beginning to be understood, a lack of consensus is surely healthy. I invited the authors to use whatever nomenclature they use within their practice, and many of them outline their rationale for their choice within their chapters. However, all of the contributors would agree that, if they choose to foreground 'abuse' in their choice of terminology, this does not mean that they exclude 'violence' from their conceptualisation, and vice versa. While the title of this book reflects this pluralism, the decision was made to use the term 'adolescent' rather than 'child' in the title, although many of the contributors refer to 'child' in their chapters. My rationale is because, in the main (although by no means exclusively), we are talking about *teenage* children who are experiencing their own social and developmental challenges at the time of the abusive behaviour. I think this developmental context is an important one to foreground, particularly given that the book's focus concerns working with families, parents and young people.

This book

A number of books have now been published on the problem of abusive behaviour towards parents. These include Price's *Power and Compassion: Working with Difficult Adolescents and Abused Parents* (Guilford Press, 1996), Cottrell's *When Teens Abuse Their Parents* (Fernwood, 2004), my own *Adolescent-to-Parent Abuse: Current Understandings in Research, Policy and Practice* (Policy Press, 2013), and Routt and Anderson's *Adolescent Violence in the Home: Restorative Approaches to Building Healthy, Respectful Family Relationships* (Routledge, 2015). There have also been some very insightful research papers and conference presentations which have explored how practitioners might start working with this problem in a range of settings and within a number of theoretical frameworks (e.g. Micucci, 1995; Sheehan, 1997; Daly and Nancarrow, 2010; Newman *et al.*, 2014). However, this is a contested field and one that is in its infancy, and the challenge of this volume is to bring together a number of practitioners and researchers of national and international standing to contribute to the debates about how best to work with adolescent abuse and violence towards parents. Many of the contributors are practitioners who have developed new ways of working, and this book draws together these exciting developments to offer guidance for practitioners, researchers and policymakers who are looking to develop their own ways of working with this problem.

The book is divided into two parts. Part 1 introduces particular therapeutic approaches to this work with contributions from practitioners whose work has been influential in shaping developments in intervention across the global North.

Its five chapters highlight a number of therapeutic approaches, and include a dual parent/young person restorative cognitive-behavioural programme known as Step-Up (Chapter 1), a solution-focused parenting support programme known as Who's in Charge? (Chapter 2), a therapeutic approach for working with parents known as non-violent resistance (NVR) (Chapter 3), a trauma and attachment-based approach to working with families (Chapter 4) and the use of systemic family therapy within a specialist filial–parental violence clinic (Chapter 5). In Part 2, the role of context in shaping practice in this field is highlighted, and these different contexts can take a number of forms. In the first three chapters, the influence of geographic and organisational contexts is highlighted, and this includes discussion of work within a mental health service in South Island, New Zealand (Chapter 6), the development of a young people's service within a domestic violence agency in London, UK (Chapter 7) and the development of a community-based intervention programme in collaboration with the local county court in Texas, USA (Chapter 8). The next two chapters examine how contexts shape experiences of and responses to this problem in terms of gender (Chapter 9) and in terms of other special considerations that might present particular challenges to the practitioner (Chapter 10). The collection concludes with a final chapter from the editor which draws together some of the common themes and debates that have emerged within the volume, and discusses the challenges that lie ahead of this exciting and important work (Chapter 11).

Notes

1 For example, such surveys may be capturing solitary violent incidents which, while not wishing to minimise their seriousness, do not form part of a wider tapestry of abuse and control. Such incidents may be less gendered than those that work to control and instil fear in another. A similar approach has been applied by Johnson (2001) in his work on types of violence found in intimate partner relationships (see Holt, 2015, for further discussion).

2 Neurodevelopmental disorders is a diagnostic category used in the current version of the *Diagnostic and Statistical Manual of Mental Disorders* (DSM-5) and includes intellectual disabilities, communication disorders, autism spectrum disorder, attention deficit hyperactivity disorder, specific learning disorder and motor disorders.

3 Indeed, such ideas have found their way into public policy across the global North. See for example the use of parental responsibility laws which ensure that parents (usually mothers) *take responsibility* for their child's offending through the use of court orders. It is regrettable that sometimes these court orders have been issued in response to cases that involved adolescent-to-parent abuse (see Holt, 2009; Condry and Miles, 2012).

References

Agnew, R. and Huguley, S. (1989). Adolescent violence towards parents. *Journal of Marriage and the Family*, *51*, 699–711.

Aroca Montolio, C., Bellver Moreno, M. C., and Alba Robles, J. L. (2013). Revision of intervention programs for the treatment of adolescent violence against parents: Guidance for the confection of a new program. *Educacion XXI*, *16*(1), 281–304.

Betancourt, N. A. (2012). *Violence from the conflict in the relations of parents and mothers with teenage children.* (Thesis, University of Colombia). Retrieved from: www.bdigital.unal.edu. co/9781/1/04870037.2012.pdf (Accessed 28 July 2014).

Boxer, P., Gullan, R. L., and Mahoney, A. (2009). Adolescents' physical aggression towards parents in a clinically referred sample. *Journal of Clinical Child and Adolescent Psychology,* *38,* 106–116.

Brezina, T. (1999). Teenage violence toward parents as an adaptation to family strain. *Youth and Society, 30*(4), 416–444.

Charles, A. V. (1986). Physically abused parents. *Journal of Family Violence, 4,* 343–355.

Christie, N. (1986). The ideal victim. In E. Fattah (ed.) *From Crime Policy to Victim Policy* (pp. 17–30). Basingstoke: Macmillan.

Condry, R. and Miles, C. (2012). Adolescent to parent violence and youth justice in England and Wales. *Social Policy and Society, 11*(2), 241–250.

Condry, R. and Miles, C. (2014). Adolescent to parent violence: Framing and mapping a hidden problem. *Criminology and Criminal Justice, Criminology and Criminal Justice, 14*(3), 257–275.

Contreras, L. and Cano, C. (2014). Family profile of young offenders who abuse their parents: A comparison with general offenders and non-offenders. *Journal of Family Violence, 29*(8), 901–910.

Cottrell, B. (2004). *When Teens Abuse their Parents.* Halifax, Nova Scotia: Fernwood.

Daly, K. and Nancarrow, H. (2010). Restorative justice and youth violence towards parents. In J. Ptacek (ed.) *Restorative Justice and Violence against Women* (pp. 150–176). Oxford: Oxford University Press.

Eckstein, N. J. (2004). Emergent issues in families experiencing adolescent-to-parent abuse. *Western Journal of Communication, 68*(4), 365–388.

Fawzi, M. H., Fawzi, M. M. and Fouad, A. A. (2013). Parent abuse by adolescents with first-episode psychosis in Egypt. *Journal of Adolescent Health, 53*(6), 730–735.

Jablonski, J. (2007). *Characteristics of parenting associated with adolescent to parent aggression.* Psy.D., Chestnut Hill College, 2007, 88 pages; AAT 3273226.

Kim J.Y., Bum, C. C. and Kyung, C. Y. (2008). The effect of domestic violence experience on adolescents' violence towards their parents and the mediating effect of the internet addiction. *Korea Social Welfare, 60*(2), 29–51.

Ghanizadeh, A. and Jafari, P. (2010). Risk factors of abuse of parents by their ADHD children. *European Child & Adolescent Psychiatry, 19*(1), 75–81.

González-Álvarez, M., Gesteira, C., Fernández-Arias, I. and García-Vera, M. P. (2010). Adolescentes que agreden a sus padres. Un análisis descriptivo de los menores agresores [Adolescents who assault their parents. A descriptive analysis of juvenile offenders]. *Psicopatología Clínica Legal y Forense, 10,* 37–53.

Goodman, L. A., Smyth, K. F., Borges, A. M. and Singer, R. (2009). When crises collide: How intimate partner violence and poverty intersect to shape women's mental health and coping. *Trauma, Violence, & Abuse, 10*(4), 306–329.

Haw, A. (2010). *Parenting over Violence: Understanding and Empowering Mothers Affected by Adolescent Violence in the Home.* Patricia Giles Centre: Perth, Australia.

Holt, A. (2009). Parent abuse: Some reflections on the adequacy of a youth justice response. *Internet Journal of Criminology,* November, 1–11. Available from: www.internetjournalof criminology.com/Holt_Parent_Abuse_Nov_09.pdf

Holt, A. (2013). *Adolescent-to-Parent Abuse: Current Understandings in Research, Policy and Practice.* Bristol: Policy Press.

Holt, A. (2015). Adolescent-to-parent abuse as a form of 'domestic violence': A conceptual review. *Trauma, Violence, & Abuse.*

Hsu, M. C., Huang, C. Y. and Tu, C. H. (2014). Violence and mood disorder: Views and experiences of adult patients with mood disorders using violence toward their parents. *Perspectives in Psychiatric Care, 50,* 111–121.

Ibabe, I., Arnoso, A. and Elgorriaga, E. (2014). Behavioral problems and depressive symptomatology as predictors of child-to-parent violence. *European Journal of Psychology Applied to Legal Context, 6*(2), 53–61.

Jackson, D. (2003) Broadening constructions of family violence: Mothers' perspectives of aggression from their children. *Child and Family Social Work, 8*(4), 321–329.

Johnson, M. P. (2001). Conflict and control: Symmetry and asymmetry in domestic violence. In A. Booth, A. C. Crouter and M. Clements (eds.) *Couples in Conflict* (pp. 95–104). Mahwah, NJ: Erlbaum.

Kennedy, T. D., Edmonds, W. A., Dann, K. T. J. and Burnett, K. F. (2010). The clinical and adaptive features of young offenders with histories of child–parent violence. *Journal of Family Violence, 25*(5), 509–520.

Laporte, L., Jiang, D., Pepler, D. J. and Chamberland, C. (2009). The relationship between adolescents' experience of family violence and dating violence. *Youth and Society, 43*(1), 3–27.

Laurent, A. and Derry, A. (1999). Violence of French adolescents toward their parents: Characteristics and contexts. *Journal of Adolescent Health, 25*(1), 21–26.

Margolin, G. and Baucom, B. R. (2014). Adolescents' aggression to parents: Longitudinal links with parents' physical aggression. *Journal of Adolescent Health, 55*(5), 645–651.

Micucci, J. A. (1995). Adolescents who assault their parents: A family systems approach to treatment. *Psychotherapy: Theory, Research, Practice and Training, 31,* 154–161.

Miettinen, R. (2014). Vicious Karin and other suicides with violent households: (Re)constructing monsters in 17th-century Swedish suicide trials. Paper presented at *Violence Against Parents in the North of Europe,* 22–24 May 2014, Joint Committee for Nordic Research Councils for the Humanities and the Social Sciences, Nordic exploratory workshops. University of Tampere, Finland.

Moffitt, T. E. (1993). Adolescence-limited and life-course-persistent antisocial behavior: A developmental taxonomy. *Psychological Review, 100*(4), 674–701

Newman, M., Fagan, C. and Webb, R. (2014). Innovations in practice: The efficacy of nonviolent resistance groups in treating aggressive and controlling children and young people: A preliminary analysis of pilot NVR groups in Kent. *Child and Adolescent Mental Health, 19,* 138–141.

Nowakowski, E. and Mattern, K. (2014). An exploratory study of the characteristics that prevent youth from completing a family violence diversion program. *Journal of Family Violence, 29*(2), 143–149.

O'Connor, R. (2007). *Who's in Charge? A Group for Parents of Violent or Beyond Control Children.* Department of Legal Studies; Faculty of Education, Humanities, Law and Theology. Flinders University, Adelaide, South Australia. Bachelor of Justice and Society.

O'Leary, K. D., Malone, J. and Tyree, A. (2004). Physical aggression in early marriage: Pre-relationship and relationship effects. *Journal of Consulting and Clinical Psychology, 62*(3), 594–602

Pagani, L. S., Tremblay, R. E., Nagin, D., Zoccolillo, M., Vitaro, M. and McDuff, P. (2004). Risk factor models for adolescent verbal and physical aggression toward mothers. *International Journal of Behavioral Development, 28*(6), 528–537.

Paulson, M. J., Coombs, R. H. and Landsverk, J. (1990). Youth who physically assault their parents. *Journal of Family Violence, 5,* 121–133.

Pearce, D. (1978). The feminization of poverty: Women, work and welfare. *Urban and Social Change Review, 11,* 28–36.

Peek, C. W., Fischer, J. L. and Kidwell, J. S. (1985). Teenage violence toward parents: A neglected dimension of family violence. *Journal of Marriage and the Family*, *47*(4), 1051–1058.

Pelletier, D. and Coutu, S. (1992). Substance abuse and family violence in adolescents. *Canada's Mental Health*, *40*(2), 6-12.

Perera, H. (2006). Parent battering and the psychiatric and family correlates in children and adolescents. *Sri Lanka Journal of Child Health*, *35*, 128–132.

Price, J. A. (1996). *Power and Compassion: Working with Difficult Adolescents and Abused Parents*. New York: Guilford Press.

Purcell, R., Baksheev, G. N. and Mullen, P. E. (2014). A descriptive study of juvenile family violence: Data from intervention order applications in a Children's Court. *International Journal of Law and Psychiatry*, *37*(6), 558–563.

Routt, G. and Anderson, L. (2011). Adolescent violence towards parents. *Journal of Aggression, Maltreatment & Trauma*, *20*(1), 1–19.

Routt, G. and Anderson, L. (2015). *Adolescent Violence in the Home: Restorative Approaches to Building Healthy, Respectful Family Relationships*. New York: Routledge.

Sheehan, M. (1997). Adolescent violence – strategies, outcomes and dilemmas in working with young people and their families. *Australian and New Zealand Journal of Family Therapy*, *18*(2), 80–91.

Shon, P. C. and Barton-Bellessa, S. M. (2012). Pre-offense characteristics of nineteenth-century American parricide offenders: An archival exploration. *Journal of Criminal Psychology*, *2*(1), 51–66.

Strom, K. J., Warner, T. D., Tichavsky, L. and Zahn, M. A. (2014). Policing juveniles: Domestic violence arrest policies, gender and police response to child–parent violence. *Crime & Delinquency*, *60*(3), 427–450

Ullman, A. and Straus, M. A. (2003). Violence by children against mothers in relation to violence between parents and corporal punishment by parents. *Journal of Comparative Family Studies*, *34*(1), 41–60.

Vink, R., Pannebakker, F., Goes, A. and Doornink, N. (2014). *Domestic violence by children and young people towards their parents: Key findings from exploratory research* [online]. Foundation Kinderpostzegels Netherlands, TNO and Movisie. Retrieved from: www.movisie.nl/publicaties/huiselijk-geweld-door-kinderen-jongeren-tegen-hun-ouders (5 February 2015).

PART 1

Therapeutic approaches

Given the complexity of adolescent violence and abuse towards parents, in terms of pathways, conceptual dilemmas and challenges in practice, it is not surprising that a range of therapeutic approaches have been proposed as vehicles for change. Each of the contributors to this section has considerable experience of working with this issue, and over time they have developed methods and techniques that work for their particular clients. Each contributor also has a unique professional background, and their training and past experience of working in related fields is also evident in the approaches they advocate. The contributors to this section have been selected because of their international standing in this field and because they each highlight different ways of thinking about and working with abuse and violence towards parents. This section comprises five chapters which outline particular theoretical approaches to this work. In Chapter 1, *Gregory Routt and Lily Anderson* discuss their dual parent–child group programme 'Step-Up'. Developed in Washington, DC, it is based on ideas from cognitive-behavioural skill-learning and restorative practice, and also draws conceptually from the influential Duluth Model used in adult IPV programs. In Chapter 2, *Eddie Gallagher* discusses his 'Who's in Charge?' approach to empowering parents. Developed in Melbourne, Australia, the programme draws on solution-focused brief therapeutic principles alongside ideas from narrative therapy, positive psychology and strengths-based approaches. In Chapter 3, *Haim Omer* discusses his development of non-violent resistance (NVR) training in Tel Aviv, Israel, to work with abused parents. NVR has its roots in the socio-political arena and draws on the principles and practices of resistance used by disadvantaged groups to fight exploitation and oppression. In Chapter 4, *Jane Evans* discusses her use of trauma-based approaches when working with young people and their families in Bristol, UK. Influenced by theory and research from neuroscience, neurobiology, attachment and trauma, Jane describes how working with past traumas can enable family members to find new ways of responding to stress and conflict. Finally, in Chapter 5, *Roberto Pereira* discusses his work based in his clinic for adolescent violence in Bilbao, Spain. Roberto describes how adopting a systemic-relational model can yield insights into seemingly irrational violent behaviours that can be used to help family members interact more peacefully.

1

BUILDING RESPECTFUL FAMILY RELATIONSHIPS

Partnering restorative practice with cognitive-behavioral skill learning

Gregory Routt and Lily Anderson

Introduction

When parents of adolescents who are violent in the home are asked what changes they would like to see their teen make, we hear different responses. Some parents immediately reply, "I want him to stop hitting me." For others the emotional abuse is more intolerable than the physical violence: "I don't want to repeat the foul names she calls me. I'm ashamed to even think she says them to anyone." Still other parents long for an end to the harassment from threats, verbal attacks, incessant demands and interminable arguing: "I try to get away from him by locking myself in my bedroom, but he yells and pounds the door for hours." Beyond the physical violence and emotional abuse, parents also have hopes of restoring a healthy relationship with their child: "I want to sit down with her to calmly talk about her grades. I want to spend time doing something fun with her, like we used to do. I want my daughter back." Parents have seemingly tried everything and feel locked in a cycle of violence with no way out. They find temporary relief when they make fewer demands on their teen, but aggression and violence return when parents reinstate clear limits. More severe consequences only lead to more abuse while parents helplessly watch their leadership slip away. When teens see their parents fail to hold boundaries, they may begin to use high-risk behaviors such as skipping school, using drugs and alcohol or violating curfews. Parents and teens also become locked in a cycle of shame. Teens feel shame when they hurt family members and fail to meet developmental milestones. Parents feel shame as they perceive themselves as inept and through stigmatization by others who see them as lax and incompetent (Edenborough *et al.*, 2008; Holt, 2011; Nixon, 2012). The cycle of shame is fed by seemingly endless rounds of anger, criticism, and blame.

We have worked exclusively with adolescent violence towards parents since 1997. Our work has included over 1,000 interviews with parents and teens and hundreds of weekly group sessions with them. These families represent a wide diversity of ethnic, religious, and socio-economic backgrounds. Teens are sometimes challenged by trauma, mental health issues, and drug and alcohol problems. Through our many years of trial and error, and learning from youth and parents, we have found certain practices especially helpful in guiding youth through a transformative process toward personal responsibility and behavioral change: parents regain leadership in their family and feel more confident parenting their youth. *Restorative practice* is one such approach. It provides a framework for intervention and a process for rebuilding healthy family relationships damaged by hurtful behavior. It emphasizes family safety and accountability for harmful behavior, and it provides a safe psychological space for everyone, providing that clearly defined boundaries are set. When used carefully, restorative practice teaches youth and parents how to talk about the violence and abuse in a meaningful and productive way. It leads youth out of cycles of violence and shame and moves them toward mutual understanding, empathy, and making amends. A second approach, *cognitive-behavioral learning and skill development*, supports the restorative process and we have found that partnership between the two is particularly effective for these families. When teens learn how to change their internal cognitive-emotional process that leads to abuse and when parents and teens practice communication and problem-solving skills together, mutual understanding and respect between them can be restored. In addition, group sessions offer a community of support that breaks feelings of isolation and shame and provides an opportunity to learn by observing others practice skills. Groups also provide a source of peer feedback and offer a community to whom participants are accountable for making behavioral changes. In this chapter, we provide an overview of Step-Up, an intervention model we developed for working with adolescent violence in the home, which partners restorative practice with cognitive-behavioral skill development. We describe its theoretical underpinnings, key components, and strategies for practice, including how we assess families to ensure they are an appropriate fit for this model. An in-depth discussion of restorative practice sheds light on how restorative principles help young people engage in accountability, develop empathy, and restore family relationships. We highlight the benefits of coupling restorative practice with cognitive-behavioral skills-based learning and how these practices mutually support each other. Finally we share some examples of group exercises that we facilitate in our group sessions.

The history of Step-Up

Our professional experience in working with adult domestic violence offenders and survivors and in parent education laid the foundation for our work with adolescent violence in the home. Lily worked with survivors of domestic violence, facilitated a parents' anger management program, authored an anger management and parenting skills curriculum for parents who were abusive with their children, and co-authored a curriculum for parents whose children witnessed domestic violence. Greg facilitated treatment groups for men who were arrested for domestic violence. We were well acquainted with the dynamics and behaviors of family and intimate partner violence, but children abusing parents was new territory. When we began our program, Step-Up, in 1997 the number of juvenile domestic violence cases in King County, Washington (USA) was staggering. Approximately 800–900 juvenile domestic violence cases were referred to the court every year; 85 percent of cases constituted violence against a family member, with 65 percent of these victims being parents. These were most often situations where a parent called the police during a violent incident by their teen. The need to address this critical issue resulted in the development of a specialized program for these young people and their parents. We knew we had a lot to learn and were faced with many unanswered questions. What dynamics are operating when a teen abuses his or her parent? When a parent is afraid of his or her teen, how is it different from intimate partner violence? Most importantly, what helps an adolescent change abusive and violent behavior? What helps a parent cope with the violence in the home? What helps a parent continue *to parent* a child she/he fears? How can we help teens and parents work together to learn respectful family relationship skills and restore their relationships? The search for answers to these questions led to some unique ways of working with these families.

Theoretical foundations

We adopted methods used by practitioners in a variety of fields which have been evaluated and shown to be effective. Within a broad framework of restorative practice, we weaved together strategies from domestic violence treatment, cognitive-behavioral therapy, anger management, solution-focused brief therapy, and family relationship skill-building – all practiced in a group setting with parents and teens. Some of the best practice and evidence-based approaches that inform our work includes:

- **Cognitive-behavioral learning and skills-based approaches** that have become the mainstay of programs that teach non-violence to children and adults (Crick & Dodge, 1994; Bandura, 1973; Lochman, Powell, Boxmeyer, Deming, & Young, 2007; Kazdin & Weisz, 1998)
- **Motivational interviewing techniques** that foster engagement of young people in the change process (Miller & Rollnick, 2002)
- **Strengths-based, solution-focused practices** that promote change by accentuating young people and their family's existing strengths and positive qualities (Clark, 1998)
- **Anger management, relaxation and self-calming techniques** that are effective in promoting the regulation of emotions (Kassinove & Tafrate, 2002)
- **Modeling positive behaviors** and giving feedback on performance (Cullen, 2002)
- **The Duluth Model tool for accountability**: specifically, the Power and Control Wheel and the Equality Wheel (Mederos, 2002; Pence & Paymar,

1993), which we have adapted for adolescent behaviors within the family and renamed as the Abuse/Disrespect and Mutual Respect Wheels.

The primary intervention goals are respect between family members and a respectful home where every person feels valued. *Respect* has universal appeal as a moral virtue valued by all religions, cultures, and classes and it operates as a moral compass for decision-making among family members – offering a standard by which all family interactions are evaluated. Respect has a synergistic effect, as Lawrence-Lightfoot (2000) contends: "Respectful relationships have a way of sustaining and replicating themselves. Respect generates respect; a modest loaf becomes many" (p. 10). When children and parents show respect for each other, as well as receive respect from each other, their mutuality strengthens and their personal confidence and self-esteem are bolstered. A culture of respect inoculates a family against hostility and aggression (Mayseless & Scharf, 2011). Helping families learn and integrate a respect template for relating to each other gives them new options for expressing themselves and responding to others in safe and respectful ways.

Our Abuse/Disrespect and Mutual Respect Wheels (Figure 1.1), adapted from the Duluth Model (Pence & Paymar, 1993), define respect in terms of actual lived behaviors. The wheels illustrate and define abuse and respect in a family and provide weekly guidance for young people with examples of specific respectful behaviors to replace the abuse and violence. Parents use the wheels to re-establish healthy boundaries with their children and to renew family relationships. The two wheels are vital to the restorative process since they join parents and young people in a mutually engaging venture to rebuild their relationship. We will describe how the wheels are also used at the beginning of each group session later in this chapter.

The structure of the program

The program utilizes a 21-session curriculum in weekly 90-minute groups where young people and their parents learn and practice skills for respectful, non-violent family relationships and safety in the home. It includes a youth group, a parent group, and a joint parent–youth group. Separate sessions for parents offer support and teach skills that enable parents to re-establish leadership. Separate sessions for teens provide them with the opportunity to learn personal skills away from their parents. Joint sessions provide opportunities for parents and young people to learn respectful communication, problem-solving and restorative skills. Young people and parents each have their own program manuals. Our sessions begin with parents and teens together for "check-in," followed by skill learning – either in separate parent and teen groups or in joint sessions, depending on the topic.

Prerequisites for the intervention

In order for a young person to be a candidate for this intervention, the assessment must demonstrate that the following criteria are fulfilled:

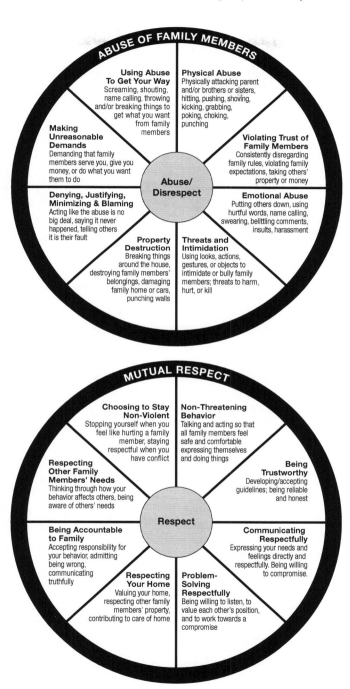

FIGURE 1.1 Abuse/Disrespect and Mutual Respect Wheels

- The young person is the **primary perpetrator** of violence in the family
- The young person's violence is **not a response to abuse**
- The young person is **not currently being abused**
- The young person has not been abused by the targeted parent(s).

If either the young person or their parents are experiencing mental health problems, then they must be **receiving appropriate treatment** for this and they must **be able to engage appropriately** in group sessions, comprehend the concepts, and learn new skills.

If either the young person or their parents have substance misuse issues, they must be **receiving recommended treatment** and must **not be currently using any addictive substances**.

Assessment of young people and families: the Behavior Checklist

Families experiencing youth violence do not fit a specific profile. Young people who are violent in the home have a variety of risk and protective factors, life experiences, and needs. A wide array of influences impacts their behavior. The common factor is that they are hurting and frightening their family members. Parents have diverse backgrounds and parenting styles. In order to determine if young people and parents are appropriate for this model, an accurate assessment of whether a family is a fit for the intervention is essential. The Behavior Checklist (Table 1.1) is an important tool used in our assessment interview.

The Behavior Checklist, administered to the teen and their parent both pre-treatment and post-treatment, identifies the teen's abusive and violent behaviors and their frequency of use. It acts as both an assessment tool for level and severity of violence and abuse, and as a measure of behavior change over the course of the intervention. It can be also be used during treatment to measure progress, serving as a motivator for behavior change. The Behavior Checklist gives a more accurate view of what is really going on and facilitates real change by providing a way to measure that change. Parents self-complete the Behavior Checklist at the intake interview and again at the end of the program. Teens fill out the same checklist about themselves.

Young people as primary aggressors in the family

While this intervention is designed for young people who are the primary perpetrators of violence in the home, young people who are being victimized by a parent and are using violence to protect themselves from being hurt by a parent do not fit this definition. In such cases, professionals are required to follow their child protection policy framework. Sometimes it is unclear who is initiating the violence. For example, parents may use violence against their child in order to protect themselves or other family members. Parents who have endured abuse for

TABLE 1.1 Behavior Checklist

Behaviors done in the last 6 months	Never	Rarely (Once)	Occasionally (Once a Month)	Frequently (Once a Week)	Almost Every Day
Called you names	1	2	3	4	5
Tried to get you to do something by intimidating you	1	2	3	4	5
Gave you angry looks or stares	1	2	3	4	5
Screamed or yelled at you	1	2	3	4	5
Threatened to hit or throw something at you	1	2	3	4	5
Pushed, grabbed or shoved you	1	2	3	4	5
Put you or other family members down	1	2	3	4	5
Threatened and/or hit brothers or sisters	1	2	3	4	5
Demanded that you or other family members do what you want	1	2	3	4	5
Said things to scare you	1	2	3	4	5
Slapped, hit, or punched you	1	2	3	4	5
Told you that you were a bad parent	1	2	3	4	5
Threw, hit, kicked, or smashed something during an argument	1	2	3	4	5
Kicked you	1	2	3	4	5

some time may respond by slapping, pushing, grabbing, or hitting in the midst of the teen's physical attack. Alternatively, a father may intervene to protect the mother and hold the son down or push him up against the wall to restrain him. In these cases, it is important to assess the risk level for harm to both parent and teen and the immediate safety issues.

Parents who contribute to their child's violence

One parent might enable a young person's abusive behavior towards the other parent. For example, a teen who visits his father – a father who had abused his mother in the past – might be given messages that serve to validate or justify his own violent behavior (for example, the mother is "crazy" or "difficult"). Some mothers report that after their child's visit with the father, the teen's abusive behavior becomes worse. These cases are particularly difficult because it is challenging for a teen to change behavior that is being supported by one of the parents.

Another way that parents contribute to their child's violence is by reacting to the abuse with physical responses. It is a challenge to stay calm when daily life involves being continually name-called and sworn at. Sometimes parents slap their teens or push them away. These are parents who regret their highly emotional reactions and want to find other ways to respond; they know they are making the situation worse and are not helping their child. In other cases, parents use violence to teach or discipline their child. Parents, especially fathers, want their child to understand that if they use violence, they will receive violence in return. In such cases, the parents' violence is not protective, but is used to stop their child's violence by overpowering them and, in some cases, inflicting physical harm. In our experience, most of these cases result in an escalation of violence in the home, and a pattern of violence between parents and youth becomes entrenched. These cases are carefully assessed and may require a report to child protection services.

Some parents may have used harsh parenting behaviors in the past (such as using a belt, yelling, put-downs, or slapping) but no longer do so. In these cases, and in those described above, the most important consideration is whether the parent can acknowledge that the behavior is/was harmful, feels remorse and is committed to no longer using such behaviors. In order for parents to regain leadership and respect, non-violence must be a family standard that everyone follows and anyone who has used violence or abuse must take responsibility for their behavior. When parents take responsibility for their violence, they are modeling accountability for their child and setting a standard for their family.

Key components of the Step-Up model

1. Safety of Family Members
   Safety in the home is a primary concern when a young person has been violent toward family members. Safety includes practices for ongoing assessment

and monitoring of risk level, safety planning, and ensuring a safe therapeutic environment. Stopping the violence and keeping a finger on the pulse of family safety are goals that shape our strategies and are always priorities.

2. Respectful Communication

    The notion of talking about difficult feelings or needs and working through disagreements while staying respectful is alien to those who have experienced violence in their families. For some people there are only two options: to express feelings or views of difficult issues in a highly emotional, blaming and aggressive way, or to avoid them altogether. Respectful communication skills are learned and practiced with the parent and teen together, where they can role-play how to talk respectfully even when angry, express feelings and needs, and solve problems while valuing each other's perspectives.

3. Understanding Cognitive, Emotive and Behavioral Processes

    Understanding the relationship between thoughts, feelings, and behavior, and taking charge of all three through self-awareness, empowers young people to change their behavior. By recognizing and understanding the feelings beneath their anger, young people learn how to move from rage to a place where they can acknowledge difficult feelings and think about how to express feelings and needs in a safe and respectful way.

4. Self-Calming and Emotional Regulation

    Most teens and parents who come to our program have lived day to day with tension between them, enduring cycles of blow-ups, remorse, and attempts to get along until another outburst sends them back to tension and high emotion. Both young people and their parents often lack the ability to calm themselves and manage emotions in the heat of conflict as well as during daily challenges. Once teens and parents learn the skill of disengaging from conflict, they can learn to self-soothe and calm the physical arousal and feelings of anger, frustration, and anxiety they are often left with as they sit in their room or walk around the block. Self-calming techniques are helpful tools to use during a difficult conversation to prevent escalation.

5. Support and Skills for Parents

    Parents often come to counseling feeling that they have lost all authority and influence with their teenager, and can no longer address issues of concern with their teen without the disruption of abuse or violence. Parents are supported in re-establishing leadership in the home by learning to safely address behavioral issues with their teen. Parents receive support from other parents and learn skills specific to parenting an adolescent who is violent toward family members.

Restorative practice

In contrast to the *retributive justice* that defines crime as an offence against the state, *restorative justice* views crime as an act that directly harms people and the community (Wachtel, 2013). Restorative practice evolved out of restorative justice, with the growing recognition that its philosophy and principles apply to areas outside the justice system, such as schools, the workplace, and families (Wachtel, 2012). In brief, restorative justice focuses on the harms resulting from an offence and helps offenders understand how their actions have affected people so they can take responsibility by doing something to repair the damage or harm. An emphasis on victims' experiences and their resulting needs acknowledges and validates the victims while offenders gain insight into the consequences of their actions. This insight enables offenders to address the causes of their behavior and develop competencies to keep them from re-offending.

However, restorative justice has its own challenges. Kathleen Daly suggests that restorative justice

> assumes that victims can be generous to those who have harmed them, that offenders can be apologetic and contrite for their behavior, that their respective "communities of care" can take an active role of support and assistance, and that a facilitator can guide rational discussion and encourage consensual decision-making between parties with antagonistic interests.
>
> (Daly, 2008: 134)

In cases of interpersonal violence, restorative justice has been criticized for perpetuating power imbalances between victims and offenders (Stubbs, 2002), often serving to re-victimize the victim and creating more fear and abuse. This is also a concern with youth-to-parent violence if the intervention is not properly structured. An analysis of restorative youth justice conferences with youth-to-parent violence in Australia found that the standard, one-time conference model "is poorly equipped and resourced to address the violence" (Daly & Nancarrow, 2008: 33).

However, restorative practice is particularly well equipped to address violence in the home when the concerns cited above *are* addressed. First, when a structured and safe environment is in place, all participants feel secure and protected so that honest and open communication is possible. Second, when everyone is learning new skills to communicate with each other, their ability to solve problems is enhanced. Third, when the process is conducted in a group setting with other families who have similar experiences, support and encouragement from participants strengthens their learning experience. Finally, restorative practice can engage young people in very profound ways. When people use violence, they morally disengage from the people they hurt and find a reason or justification for their behavior (Bandura *et al.*, 1996). Young people are often unaware of the repercussions on their parents' lives and the lives of others, such as siblings, who are impacted by their behavior. Restorative practice attempts to evoke moral emotions, such as guilt, empathy, sympathy, and compassion, by helping young people to understand the harm they have caused to another person. Indeed, young people are more inclined to feel empathy and remorse after hurting family members, as opposed to a peer or a stranger.

Reducing shame through restorative process

Hurting a family member evokes emotions such as shame and guilt, which can interfere with accountability, empathy, and behavior change. When people feel ashamed of themselves they are less motivated to take responsibility – instead, they deny their actions, withdraw, and avoid people. They may become hostile and angry at the world: "In short, shamed individuals are inclined to assume a defensive posture, rather than take a constructive, reparative stance in their relationships" (Tangney & Dearing, 2002: 180–181). These are the very behaviors many parents describe in their child when they come to us for help. Therefore, a key element of restorative practice is to reduce shame by reframing the wrongdoing as the behavior, not the person. It is the difference between *who I am* and *what I did*, or "self" versus "behavior" (Tangney & Dearing, 2002: 24). In their book *Shame and Guilt* (2002), Tangney and Dearing describe how there are good ways to feel bad about wrongdoing and ways that are not so good. They believe shame and guilt are two very different emotions and shape a person's perspective of his or her wrongdoing. Put simply, shame is self-focused while guilt is behavior-focused. Shame is a negative evaluation of the self, while guilt is a negative evaluation of behavior. They explain how shame appears to be the less "moral" emotion, explaining that when people feel ashamed of themselves they are less motivated to take responsibility and make things right. Guilt, on the other hand, has a more adaptive function since "[it] causes us to stop and re-think – and it offers a way out, pressing us to confess, apologize, and make amends" (Tangney & Dearing, 2002: 180). When shame is lifted, there is a greater capacity for empathy. When one opens to feelings of empathy, it ignites a sense of personal responsibility and a need to do something to help the person harmed or "make it right" in some way. It is at this point in the process where it is especially important for adolescents to experience encouragement and support. As feelings of empathy arise, they are vulnerable to slipping back into shame, shutting off the empathy and disengaging from the process.

The key to this process is allowing young people to experience the discomfort of their difficult feelings as they recognize the impact of their behavior, while helping them feel supported and competent. It is here where adolescents often "jump ship" as feelings become uncomfortable and they go back to blaming others. This may also be when both parents and professionals become uncomfortable and want to protect the young person from difficult feelings. Helping young people feel safe and supported while they experience uncomfortable feelings helps them to learn that they can have difficult emotions without withdrawing from or attacking others. When young people are allowed to feel the disquiet of having hurt their family members, they begin to feel internally motivated to do something about it. This leads them to the next step in the process: accountability for behavior through reparative acts. Taking active accountability further reduces their shame by increasing their self-respect.

Accountability: transforming shame into self-respect

When adolescents take active responsibility for their behavior, whether it is repairing a hole in the wall or doing chores to make money to replace a broken lamp, their shame is transformed into feeling capable. Making amends gives teens an opportunity to regain their dignity and self-respect. They feel competent when they are able to do something about what has happened, as opposed to walking around carrying self-blame and shame, and often coping with their difficult feelings by blaming others. Blame is a means to convince themselves and others that their behavior was justified and that they are not a bad person; there is a reason for the behavior. When teens have another way to show others and themselves that they really are "good" by doing something to make things right, such as showing kindness for the person or helping them, their sense of self is lifted. In our experience with young people, we often see a shift once they have actively taken steps to make amends. This is usually when the teen takes a significant step forward in the change process, becoming more engaged and hopeful.

Restorative principles

Restorative practice is guided by the following principles, which promote engagement and investment in successful outcomes. These principles are central to helping young people who are violent in the family move from an external motivation to an internal motivation to change. They set the stage to support learning – whether it is cognitive-behavioral understanding or skill-building – in a way that supports and respects young people:

- *Respect for all* proposes that all sides in a conflict must be listened to and that every person is valued, respected, and has the opportunity to be heard
- *Collaborative problem-solving* obliges all parties in a conflict to work together to find a solution
- *Fair process* means all participants must feel that they are treated fairly. When a person is challenged for doing something wrong, it is in a firm but fair manner. The person's point of view is included in the process and expectations are clearly explained with input from all who are involved.

Working "with" young people

There are four approaches to addressing wrongdoing:

1. A punitive approach of doing things *to* the person
2. A neglectful approach of *not* responding
3. A permissive approach of doing things *for* the person
4. A restorative approach of working *with* the person to facilitate positive change.

This is not a new concept, and is often used by parent educators to describe different styles of parenting. Restorative practice relies on the working "with" approach to engage and guide people through the change process. This approach is particularly useful with teenagers, who quite often have not volunteered to participate in an intervention to address their violence. Most of our young people have been externally motivated to attend the program, by the court or by their parents. Guiding them from external to internal motivation is the most important work we do.

Figure 1.2 depicts the four approaches of addressing wrongdoing, developed by Ted Wachtel from the International Institute for Restorative Practice.[1] Two axes support the window: the vertical axis represents the level of *social control* exerted on a person and the horizontal axis represents the level of *support* offered to a person. *Low social control* includes vague or absent behavioral standards and rules that lack consequences and accountability if violated. *High social control* involves explicit boundaries and expectations regarding behavioral standards, along with consistent responses to violations. The level of *support* ranges from *high support*, in which guidance and assistance are provided, to *low support*, where there is minimal help, concern, or encouragement.

The punitive approach is *high in control*, but *low in support*, offering less social or emotional incentive for change, leaving fear of punishment done *to* the person as the only motivator to make change. The permissive approach is *high in support*, but tends to rescue and protect the person from consequences. The neglectful approach, with *low control* and *low support*, leaves the person alone, without incentive or support for change. The restorative *with* approach, with *high support* and *high control*, provides a balance of what is needed for young people to make change – clear boundaries and behavioral expectations, consequences that help them take responsibility for their behavior when they go off the path, and support and

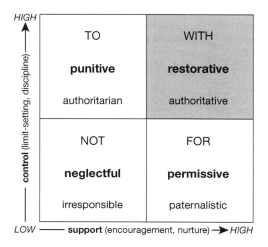

FIGURE 1.2 Approaches to addressing wrongdoing

encouragement to help them feel competent to make change. In sum, the restorative approach we advocate involves a balance of *accountability for behavior* and *support for making change.*

Restorative inquiry

A set of questions (see Table 1.2) enable *restorative inquiry* and are used to guide the person who has exhibited harmful behavior through a process that is the "essence of restorative justice" (Zehr, 2002: 38). The questions are designed to engage the person to reflect on the effects of the harmful behavior on others, experience empathy, and take responsibility for the harm that was caused by making amends. When a young person has been violent toward a family member during the previous week, we ask him or her to read and respond to the following restorative questions from the perspective of the parent. The parent can then describe and clarify his or her experience.

Check-in: accountability, behavior change and restoring relationships

Every group opens with *check-in.* Teens use the Abuse and Respect Wheels in their reflections on their previous week and how they behaved. Parents give their perspective, adding "respectful" or "abusive" behaviors that they feel are significant and were not reported by the teens. If a young person has been physically violent or has threatened physical violence during the previous week, they answer the restorative inquiry questions (described above) with input from the parent. During check-in, teens also report on their progress with their behavior change plan, or what we call their "goal for the week." Young people evaluate the extent to which they met the previous week's goal and they then set a goal for the following week. For example, if they were physically violent during the previous week, their goal would be an action they intend to take to prevent further physical violence. Teens complete a series of questions on a worksheet that helps them think through how they will meet the goal. They identify respectful behaviors that they will substitute for the abusive ones.

Check-in serves a number of purposes for teens, parents, and group facilitators. Teens are held accountable to the group for their behavior and for meeting specific personal goals. Check-in also offers young people an opportunity to evaluate their progress toward using more respectful behaviors. It also provides positive reinforcement from the group as well as their parents for using respectful behaviors at home. Weekly check-in using the Abuse and Respect Wheels raises young people's awareness of their behavior at home during the week. When they know they will be reporting to the group about their behaviors, they are incentivized to practice more respectful behaviors. Young people tell us that check-in helps them pay attention to their behavior. Some parents say that they believed check-in was the most influential group exercise in helping their child change.

Parents learn to reframe their perspectives on their teens' hurtful behaviors. Instead of simply responding with anger and criticism, parents learn to evaluate behavior based on whether it was respectful or disrespectful. This allows them to talk about hurtful behavior with their child in a different way. They learn to notice

TABLE 1.2 Questions for restorative inquiry

Restorative inquiry

	Question	*Rationale*
1	**Who was harmed by my behavior?** Who else in my family was affected by my behavior?	These questions help the young person think about all of the people who were affected in some way by the behavior. It helps them to recognize the larger impact of their behavior.
2	**What was the harm, damage, or loss resulting from the hurtful behavior?** How did my behavior affect each person? How did it affect our relationship? How did the behavior cause a problem?	These questions help the young person to understand the impact of their behavior from other people's perspective. They activate empathy and help young people to begin to feel a sense of responsibility for their behavior.
3	**How did it affect me?** How do I feel about how I handled the situation? What were the negative consequences for me?	These questions help the young person to recognize that they are also impacted negatively by their violent or abusive behavior.
4	**In this situation what could I have done differently?** What other respectful choices did I have for how to respond? Are there any behaviors on the Respect Wheel that I could have used? What skills could I have used? How could I have expressed my feelings or needs in a respectful way?	These questions remind young people that behavior is a choice and that they have other options for responding to anger. This helps them think through and remember the skills they are learning for non-violent, respectful responses.
5	**How can I make amends?** What do I need to do to repair the harm or problems caused? What can I do to address the needs of those harmed and make amends? What do I need to do to begin to repair the relationship?	These questions helps the young person to learn that true accountability means taking responsibility for harm caused by their behavior and taking steps to repair the damage. They begin to understand the meaning of making amends in their relationship.
6	**What is my plan to prevent me from repeating the behavior?** What specifically will I do the next time this situation arises? What might get in the way of behaving in a new way and what should I do to prevent that?	We close with having them make a specific behavioral plan to prevent using the behavior again.

and acknowledge respectful behavior – thus reinforcing the use of respect in the home for the entire family. For facilitators, check-in provides a way to measure teens' progress, identify particular problem behaviors, and tailor specific strategies for each young person. When a teen has difficulty meeting a weekly goal, the facilitator can invite suggestions from other group members. The facilitator encourages parents to acknowledge the respectful behaviors their teens used during the week and reminds them of their strengths and ability to choose respectful behaviors. Facilitators play an important modeling role in demonstrating how parents might talk to teens about abusive behavior and acknowledge their child's competencies. Finally, facilitators can identify specific parent–teen dynamics that might be barriers to progress.

Thinking, beliefs, and feelings: how they work together to influence behavior

Once young people begin to understand the impact of their behavior on others and experience empathy through the restorative process, they begin to feel internal motivation to change. Cognitive-behavioral learning gives them the skills for changing their hurtful behavior and sustaining respectful family relationships. Helping teens become aware of how their thoughts, feelings, and beliefs interact with and influence their actions raises self-awareness and insight about what is happening internally for them when they become aggressive. As facilitators, we explore how people's perceptions and thinking about a situation impact on how they feel and react, and even more importantly, how perceptions and thinking can be inaccurate. Teens learn how changing the way they think about a situation can calm or shift negative feelings so these feelings become less intense. Teaching teens how to slow down and observe how their cognitive, emotive, and behavioral processes leads to hurtful behavior provides information that can help them change their response. Likewise, looking at their cognitive processes when they choose non-violent, respectful responses informs them about their ability to steer their course in a positive direction by thinking and believing in more helpful ways.

This cognitive-behavioral segment of the intervention includes four sessions:

1   Understanding Thinking and Self-Talk
2   Understanding Beliefs
3   Understanding Feelings
4   Putting it All Together: Changing Hurtful Moves into Helpful Moves.

The concepts learned from these sessions are integrated within the entire intervention so that they are continually reinforced and applied to current situations in the young people's lives. These four sessions support the goals of restorative practice by offering teens a way to learn how to make choices that are based on mutual respect and trust.

The role of the juvenile justice system

One of the greatest challenges for parents and professionals in this work is engaging young people who refuse intervention. Many young people are unwilling to attend counseling and parents have limited influence with a teen who is violent toward them. When there is physical violence by a teen in the home and he or she refuses help, the juvenile justice system can be a vital source of support for the family: it may be the only way to engage the young person in changing violent behavior. In addition, when there is involvement from the juvenile justice system it sends an important message to the teen: violence in the family is not acceptable. When young people are continually violent toward family members without a police or court response, they learn that violence is not a crime and is acceptable, as long as it is within the family. Violence in most schools is swiftly responded to, with zero tolerance polices clearly in place and applied to all students. Unfortunately, violence is taken less seriously when it is directed toward family members.

It helps young people to experience a response to their violence from the larger community, not just from their parents. In our experience, many teens regard their court experience as helpful to them, often citing their arrest or a few days in detention as a motivator for them to change. They benefit from the recognition that it is not only their parents who are worried; the larger community is also concerned about their behavior and the safety of their family members. It helps parents feel supported when others, such as a police officer or a judge, tell their child that the behavior is not safe and is worthy of attention from the court and the helping professionals. It is important to find out how your court system handles these cases so you can provide accurate information to families. When the court allows young people to avoid legal charges by engaging in an intervention program, parents feel more comfortable with court intervention.

However, the intervention we described in this chapter is more effective if it is part of a coordinated, community-wide effort to end violence in the home. The Duluth Model pioneered a community response to domestic violence when they created a coherent philosophical approach that prioritized victim safety, developed best practice policies for intervention agencies, reduced fragmentation in the court system's response, built a system of monitoring offenders, raised awareness of the harm domestic violence does to children, and fostered a supportive community infrastructure (Mederos, 2002). From our experience, when law enforcement officers, juvenile courts, and community agencies work together toward common goals, family safety is enhanced.

Summary

Helping adolescents change violent behavior in the home requires a multifaceted approach. It calls for bringing together practices that engage young people in self-reflection, empathy, and accountability, along with competency development that equips teens and their parents with new skills. We have found the partnership of restorative practice and cognitive-behavioral skills-based learning in a group setting to be a potent model to help youth and parents restore respectful, healthy relationships. The Step-Up approach has been evaluated showing lower recidivism rates than comparison groups, significantly reduced violence and abuse in the home, and significant improvement in youths' and parents' attitudes, skills, and behaviors over the course of the intervention (Routt & Anderson, 2011).

Note

1   See www.iirp.edu/

References

Bandura, A. (1973). *Aggression: A social learning analysis.* Englewood Cliffs, NJ: Prentice-Hall.

Bandura, A., Barbaranelli, C., Caprara, G. V., & Pastorelli, C. (1996). Mechanisms of moral disengagement in the exercise of moral agency. *Journal of Personality and Social Psychology*, 71 (2), 364–374.

Clark, M. D. (1998). Strengths-based practice: The ABC's of working with adolescents who don't want to work with you. *Federal Probation Quarterly*, 62 (1), 46–53.

Crick, N. R. & Dodge, K. A. (1994). A review and reformulation of social information-processing mechanisms in children's social adjustment. *Psychological Bulletin*, 115, 74–101.

Cullen, F. T. (2002). Rehabilitation and treatment programs. In J. Q. Wilson & J. Petersilia (eds.) *Crime: Public policy for crime control* (2nd ed.) (pp. 253–289). Oakland, CA: ICS Press.

Daly, K. (2008). The limits of restorative justice. In D. Sullivan & L. Tifft (eds.) *The handbook of restorative justice* (pp. 134–146). New York: Routledge.

Daly, K. & Nancarrow, N. (2008). Restorative justice and youth violence toward parents. In J. Ptacek (ed.) *Feminism, restorative justice, and violence against women.* New York: Oxford University Press.

Edenborough, M., Jackson, D., Mannix, J., & Wilkes, L. M. (2008). Living in the red zone: the experience of child-to-mother violence. *Child and Family Social Work*, 13, 464–473.

Holt, A. (2011). 'The terrorist in my home': teenagers' violence towards parents – constructions of parent experiences in public online message boards. *Child and Family Social Work*, 16 (4), 454–463.

Kassinove, H. & Tafrate, R. C. (2002). *Anger management: The complete treatment guidebook for practitioners.* Atascadero, CA: Impact.

Kazdin, A. E. & Weisz, J. R. (1998). Identifying and developing empirically supported child and adolescent treatments. *Journal of Consulting and Clinical Psychology*, 66, 19–36.

Lawrence-Lightfoot, S. (2000). *Respect: An exploration.* Cambridge, MA: Perseus Books.

Lochman, J., Powell, N., Boxmeyer, C., Deming, A. M., & Young, L. (2007). Cognitive-behavior group therapy for angry and aggressive youth. In R. W. Christner, J. Stewart, & P. A. Freeman (eds.) *Handbook of cognitive-behavioral group therapy with children and adolescents* (pp. 333–348). New York: Routledge.

Mayseless, O. & Scharf, M. (2011). Respecting others and being respected can reduce aggression in parent-child relations and in schools. In P. R. Shaver & M. Mikulincer (eds.) *Human aggression and violence: Causes, manifestations, and consequences* (pp. 277–294). Washington, DC: American Psychological Association.

Mederos, F. (2002). Changing our visions of intervention – the evolution of programs for physically abusive men. In E. Aldarondo & F. Mederos (eds.) *Programs for men who batter* (pp. 1–23). Kingston, NJ: Civic Research Institute.

Miller, W. R. & Rollnick, S. (2002). *Motivational interviewing* (2nd edn.). New York: Guilford.

Nixon, J. (2012). Practitioners' constructions of parent abuse. *Social Policy & Society*, 11 (2), 229–239.

Pence, E. & Paymar, M. (1993). *Education groups for men who batter: The Duluth Model*. New York: Springer.

Routt, G. & Anderson, L. (2011). Adolescent violence towards parents. *Journal of Abuse, Maltreatment and Trauma*, 20, 1–19.

Stubbs, J. (2002). Domestic violence and women's safety: Feminist challenges to restorative justice. In H. Strang & J. Braithwaite (eds.) *Restorative justice and family violence* (pp. 42–61). Melbourne: Cambridge University Press.

Tangney, J. P. & Dearing, R. L. (2002). *Shame and guilt*. New York: Guilford Press.

Wachtel, T. (2012). What is restorative practice? [online]. *International Institute for Restorative Practices*. Retrieved from www.iirp.edu/what-is-restorative-practices.php

Wachtel, T. (2013). Defining restorative [online]. *International Institute for Restorative Practices*. Retrieved at www.iirp.edu/what-is-restorative-practices.php

Zehr, H. (2002). *The little book of restorative justice*. Intercourse, PA: Good.

2

EMPOWERING PARENTS

The *Who's in Charge?* program

Eddie Gallagher

Introduction

In 1992, I was working as a family therapist in a small welfare organisation on the outskirts of Melbourne, Australia. By chance I was working simultaneously with four lone mothers who were victims of overt aggression from their sons, aged between 11 and 13. I remember a 'light-bulb moment' when I realised I was hearing the same things from, and saying the same things to, all four mothers. In my previous 18 years of therapeutic work with families I had not identified violence towards parents as an issue. I can recall three families where there had been violence directed at parents but these had come at 5-year intervals and they had little in common. I didn't conceptualise this as 'family violence' but as a child behaviour problem. I did not think of the boys' behaviour as 'abuse'. Abuse meant 'violence plus power', so how could a powerless child abuse a powerful parent? Despite my confusion about the power issues, I assumed that *empowering* the parents would be useful and decided to get the mothers together as a mini support group. All four were enthusiastic and we were soon joined by a fifth mother, who was being beaten by her 15-year-old daughter. We called it the 'MAAD' group, for 'Mothers Against Adolescent Domination'. It was purely a support group as I had little idea about what would or would not work in such situations and could find no literature with any practical advice, nor anyone with experience of the issue. The few existing research studies were more confusing than enlightening as they were full of glaring contradictions with no consensus, not even on such basic questions as gender. Many studies appeared to overtly *blame the parent* and their findings were very different from my own professional experience. Surveys of adult family violence were also radically different from my experience of working with families where there was *intimate partner violence* (IPV). I had facilitated men's behaviour change groups for many years and my approach to the issue of *child-to-parent violence* (CPV) became an amalgam of work on parenting issues and work with abusers and survivors of IPV.

Over the next few years I observed a steady stream of families where children were violent or otherwise 'abusive'. I resisted using the term 'abuse' for some time: I saw abuse as hurtful or coercive behaviour *plus power* and it felt wrong to be referring to children as 'abusers'. I counselled the young people as well as their parents, and often met siblings and other relatives. I found the majority of these parents to be caring and child-focused. Many were intelligent and more were middle-class than I would have expected. I also work with abusive parents and they seemed to be *less* likely to be targeted by their children – the opposite of the conclusion of many quantitative studies which have identified parent–child violence as mutual (e.g. Straus *et al.* 1980; Brezina 1999; Browne and Hamilton 1998). The impression from most of the literature, at least from surveys, was that parents were to blame and that they had often been violent or controlling towards their child. In contrast, clinical studies, and most qualitative studies, were framed in a way that was far more sympathetic towards the parents and did not identify them as being abusive. My *ad hoc* clinical sample, collected over 22 years from a range of referral sources (two family welfare agencies, two community health services, private practice and group programmes) now stands at 435 young people. In terms of the socio-demographic characteristics of the families I work with, there is a general ratio of two boys to one girl as instigators of parental violence, with mothers far more likely to be abused than fathers, and likely to suffer more, both physically and psychologically. However, while gender is clearly of *great* importance in CPV, I do not see it as being as *central* a factor as it is in IPV: half of all families in my sample (51 per cent) have either a girl as aggressor or a father as victim and, although a boy abusing a lone mother after IPV is the most common scenario, these still represent only a quarter of all cases in my client group. Lone parents tend to be over-represented, and there is a tendency towards formally educated, middle-class families in my client group.

Theoretical foundations and parent-blaming

My interest in child-to-parent violence has made me acutely aware of the ubiquity of *parent-blaming*. Psychology, psychiatry, social work, criminology and family therapy (more subtly) are steeped in a culture of parent-blaming. This has been primarily mother-blaming, and father-blaming can be seen as a recent development. Parent-blaming is so often taken for granted that most people are not aware of it (Caplan and Hall-McCorquodale 1985). For the second half of the last century, 'nurture' was seen as all-important and 'nature' pushed to the side, especially in clinical practice. '*Nurture*' is an unfortunate term for environmental influence since mothers are assumed to be doing the *nurturing* and the huge contribution of the wider environment is minimised, with parenting assumed to be the main component of the environment during childhood. When I was studying and working with families in the 1970s and 1980s it was almost taboo to suggest that a child's behavioural problems had anything to do with their personality. Personality was only seen as relevant if it could be fitted into an identifiable condition such as ADHD,[1] in which case parenting was then often assumed to be of little or no importance. Such naive dichotomising is still quite common.

In CPV our tendency towards parent-blaming coincides with a propensity for victim-blaming. Victim-blaming in IPV has reduced greatly over the past few decades (though it remains an issue) but attitudes to CPV are about thirty years behind and victim-blaming is still the norm. Both my therapeutic practice and the *Who's in Charge?* group have been greatly influenced by solution-focused and narrative approaches in family therapy, positive psychology and the strengths-based approach in social work. I don't follow any of these approaches dogmatically and see them all as closely related. To me, these approaches are largely common sense, partly designed to counter the negativity and client-stigmatisation inherent in more traditional approaches such as psychotherapy and the medical model of mental health.

Counselling practice

I have counselled several hundred families where there is CPV. I work directly with the young person when they will engage (many won't), with their parent or parents, and just occasionally with entire families or even extended families. I am cautious about working with entire families, or even with teenagers alongside the parents they are abusing. In adult family violence, it has long been considered bad practice to see victim and victimiser together and some of the same problems can arise in CPV if attempting to see parent and child together while there is active violence or abuse. Both parties may minimise the child's behaviour; verbal aggression may escalate within the therapy session; the aggressor may take the opportunity to verbally attack the victim and rehearse their excuses; the aggressor may feel victimised and 'got-at' and refuse to return; and the aggressor may seek revenge on the victim after the session. Therefore, my usual preference is to meet with the parent and child separately until some progress has been made. Involving other siblings in the early stages can often be counter-productive as the aggressive child will feel 'picked-on' and scapegoated. At least initially, siblings may need separate therapy.

When I work with a young person I am attempting to increase their responsibility. I use *solution-focused questioning* to encourage the responsible, caring side of their nature – which is almost always apparent to others if not to their victimised parent (Gallagher 2004b). Usually, and ideally, I work simultaneously with their parent(s) and aim to empower them to be more firm and consistent (Gallagher 2004a). If I can facilitate some change in two parts of the family system then positive feedback often comes into play and dramatic improvements can result from fairly small behavioural changes. In most cases, I consider the work with the parent to be more important and useful than the work with the child. I often state that in counselling we work with the *solution* not the *problem*, hence it is logical to work with the most motivated part of the system, and *potentially* the parent has more power than the child. I thus view parent groups as well suited to the prevention and treatment of CPV.

The *Who's in Charge?* group program

Ten years passed between the MAAD group and developing the *Who's in Charge?* group for parents. *Who's in Charge?* is a structured program comprising nine sessions which makes much use of handouts and exercises (including a few homework exercises). It has been run over one hundred times, in Australia and in the UK, and it appears to work with a variety of demographics and different cultural groups. The use of handouts means that it is somewhat more effective with more formally educated parents but we have also had success with parents with few literacy skills or where English is a second language. There are two other such parenting programmes in Victoria, Australia (Breaking the Cycle – see Paterson & Luntz 2002 and TARA (Teenage Aggression Responding Assertively) run by Berry Street). Parent groups have a number of advantages in dealing with CPV:

1 They are not expensive: in most agencies a few interested practitioners have been able to implement the program without any additional funding and after only a few days' training
2 They do not stigmatise the young person
3 They can reach those families where the young person refuses to cooperate with professionals
4 They can reach families early in the development of CPV before involvement with the legal system and before the young person becomes at serious risk of educational failure, crime, substance misuse or homelessness
5 It is enjoyable for both practitioners and parents.

Rather than describing the *Who's in Charge?* group in detail here, I will highlight some issues of general interest:

The three-part structure of the group

The first three or four sessions aim to change parental attitudes and, in particular, to reduce blame and shame. We use a variety of exercises to deconstruct some of the unhelpful myths that parents have absorbed about their child's behaviour. We aim to help them understand that children's bad behaviour is multi-causal, and we explore the nature of abuse, styles of parenting, social changes that make CPV more likely and ideas about entitlement and power. The second part of the group explores the use of *consequences* to change unwanted behaviour. This has similarities to the content of mainstream parenting groups (and advice books) but there are important differences. Most parenting advice assumes that children are cooperative. However, the parents attending *Who's in Charge?* groups typically have children who have stopped cooperating, who often appear to care about very little, who may deliberately sabotage parents' attempts to apply *consequences*, and who may escalate their violence when parents implement behavioural control strategies. In the group we explore the difficulty of identifying *consequences* that the parent can implement, is willing to control and that the child will care about (at least a little). We do not see the application of consequences in terms of *behaviour modification* but in terms of *empowerment of the parent*: increasing the child's respect for the parent, enabling the parent to be more assertive and altering the balance of positives and negatives that the young person experiences from their violent and controlling behaviour.

The third part of the group supports parents to make changes within the home while working on a few advanced topics: anger, assertiveness and self-care. The order of these topics is important. Until parents have made some attitude changes and become more empowered they are not usually ready to work on these topics. The anger topic is about *their* anger as well as understanding and dealing with the young person's anger. However, parents may not be ready to admit to, or work on, their own inappropriate behaviour early in the group process.

Thus, the structure of the group aims first to support and empower, second to encourage practical changes (usually in terms of rules and consequences) and third to reinforce these changes and cover some advanced topics. There is a steady reduction in content during the course of the group – the ideal being that groups become more positive and helpful and thus discussion increases and facilitator-directed exercises reduce.

Guilt and shame

> Blaming our mothers is so easy that we rarely stop to consider whether anyone else might be to blame, or even that no-one is to blame. For us mothers, understanding how mother-blaming operates can lighten our load.
>
> (Caplan 1998: 128)

Given the rampant parent-blaming in our culture, it is no surprise that parents abused by their children often feel intense, and sometimes immobilising, guilt. This is not just a result of them being victimised by their child but they often feel victimised by those around them, to whom they look for support and who often work within the very organisations that are meant to help them. Guilt and shame (not the same but often overlapping) are serious obstacles to parents forming working alliances with professionals. Research into CPV in a number of countries has found that parents feel blamed and feel that services are often less than helpful (Omer 2000; Eckstein 2002; Cottrell 2004; Bonnick 2006; Holt 2013).

I also consider parental guilt to play an important part in the origin and ongoing dynamics of CPV. Parental hesitancy and lack of assertion is often partly the result of guilt. When working with parents I often find that their level of assertiveness is key to turning the situation around. This is not to say that these parents are all weak and unassertive, but I do believe that many abused parents have been somewhat permissive and insufficiently firm with their children but this need not be to an extreme degree. The process whereby CPV develops is often a slow and insidious one, where the balance of power slowly shifts as children lose respect and parents slowly give ground, trying in vain to keep the peace. There are insidious circular processes within the family as the child increasingly develops defiance and aggression and the parent becomes disempowered. Denying that some children are inherently more 'difficult' than others inevitably leads to parent-blaming. Even in those families where there has been IPV, its effect on children of differing temperaments can vary dramatically. In the same family with similar exposure to a father's violence, one child may be withdrawn and nervous, another responsible and protective, another apparently unaffected and a fourth aggressive, defiant and disrespectful. Families without a past history of IPV (52 per cent of my sample) are quite likely to have other children who are well within the 'normal' range for behaviour and are often academically and socially successful. It is my belief that the same child-focused, indulgent parenting that can result in CPV is positive for children of easy or 'normal' temperaments but can backfire with a strong-willed and challenging child. The model of good parenting that has been pushed by parenting experts in recent years does not sufficiently take children's variability into account and this is the model that most practitioners also attempt to apply. A parent who has been highly child-focused and has lavished praise and attention on a child up until they rebel in adolescence may be encouraged to give that child more attention. Several parents have told me that attempting to give more attention made the child's behaviour even worse. This is not to say that the *right kind* of attention may not work well, as exemplified by the approach of Haim Omer (see Chapter 3 in this volume, or Omer 2000). One problem is that in the welfare and mental health services there is often a focus on parents who do *not* give children sufficient attention or who are neglectful or abusive. What we encourage with these parents may be insulting or counter-productive when we attempt to apply it to most parents being abused by their children.

Challenging parental guilt

> Their parents are overwhelmed by fear, anger and guilt. Guilt can be the most devastating emotion, for it often paralyses parents so that they are unable to take effective action.
>
> (Samenow 1989: 13)

Parents are frequently so mired in guilt and self-blame that this must be tackled before they can make effective use of any strategies. It is almost impossible to be assertive with someone if you are feeling intensely guilty about their behaviour (as well as feeling sorry for them and protective towards them). Thus parents are often not ready to use practical strategies until they feel empowered and become more determined. We avoid suggesting strategies in the first few sessions. This frustrates some desperate parents (though they will pick up ideas from other parents during this time). It is *vital* that facilitators believe that parents are not inevitably to blame for their children's behaviour. A recommended book to challenge the myth of the all-powerful parent is *The Nurture Assumption* (Harris 1998). The idea of parents being *largely responsible* for how their children turn out is a deep and persistent myth and most of us have been trained and acculturated into this belief over a number of years. This is not to say that inadequate parenting cannot have a profound effect on children's development and it is far easier to be a bad influence than a good influence. Challenging guilt begins in the very first group session (or during pre-group contact) with the way we talk to parents and the way we talk about the issue of CPV. Just having contact with a group of other parents is itself helpful in reducing guilt (though not sufficient) as it becomes apparent that the others are not abusive or neglectful parents.

An apparent paradox with this program is that we spend the first few sessions helping parents realise that they are only one of many influences on their child and that they may be quite limited in what influence they have. We then spend the rest of the group encouraging them to change their behaviour, rather than focusing on the need for their child to change, so as to use what influence they have in the most effective way. Work both with parents who are abused and with their children needs a balance of support and challenge. Omer states this neatly:

> Challenge and support are thus the two sides of the same coin: the more forceful our empathic endorsement of the parents' pain, values and achievements, the greater our ability to contest their ineffective behavior.
>
> (Omer 2000: 36)

Possible solutions to CPV, such as more consistent consequences for unacceptable behaviour, or even a legal order, may actually backfire unless parents are ready to firmly and assertively follow through. A planned schedule of consequences will not work if the parent is unsure, lacking in assertiveness or unprepared for their child's determined attempts to undermine them (stubborn children often get worse before they get better). For example, a parent persuaded to take out a legal order prematurely is unlikely to call the police when the child breaches the order and the child may end up feeling *more* powerful.

An exercise designed to reduce parental guilt is called Influences on Your Child, which is a core element of the *Who's in Charge?* group. The exercise is one that can be confusing, so it is fully explained in the group. We first ask, 'If your influence on your child is 10 points, how much influence has the other parent had on the same scale?' This is an arbitrary 10 points, which logically represents one unit of influence, not 10 per cent or 10 out of 10. Interestingly, mothers in intact families frequently say their partner has the same influence as themselves i.e. 10 points. Mothers with abusive ex-partners frequently say their ex-partner has twice as much influence as them i.e. 20 points. Whether such numbers are realistic or not is not the issue: it is a subjective exercise, rather than a psychometric test. We then ask in turn about (and often discuss) other influences, including step-parents, siblings, other relatives, schools, peers, media, temperament, specific events and the child's own choices. We do not include the wider culture in which the family is embedded because, while this is a vitally important influence on a child, individuals are generally unaware of this. (It is a rare fish who knows he's wet: even the influence of media is difficult for many parents to see because it is so ubiquitous in their own and their children's lives.) Once all these influences are given numerical values by each parent they are added and the percentage influence of the parent is worked out (a table simplifies this process). I have performed this exercise with hundreds of parents of aggressive children and also with about a thousand professionals who have attended my training workshops. When their individual influence is compared to the total influences on their child it typically comes out at around 10 per cent. It is very rare for anyone to score over 20 per cent except for a very young child. A low score is not necessarily problematic: a teenager with good social networks, lots of interests and a strong personality will have a parent with a low score for their perceived influence. The question we then ask parents, particularly mothers, is: 'Why are you taking all the responsibility?'

> Why are women given – and more importantly, why do women take – all the rap, when it is virtually impossible to pinpoint any one factor in a child's life that determines what that child becomes?
>
> (Jeffers 1999: 128)

This exercise makes some professionals uneasy. A few feel that suggesting that mothers are not all-important is heresy. There is also a concern that some parents might give up in despair. This does not happen in the context of CPV but I would not use this exercise with neglectful or abusive parents who would find it reassuring in an unhelpful way (and they would also underestimate their negative influence). A few parents have found the exercise upsetting because the exercise can illustrate to them that they are currently having very little influence on their beyond-control child (under 5 per cent). Although upsetting, admitting this can be a first step towards making realistic decisions. On the whole the majority of parents have found the exercise liberating and I've had parents mention it much later as a turning point.

More generally, in the first few group sessions we attempt to counter 'pat' explanations for children's aggressive or abusive behaviour. Some parents have simplistic ideas about there being *one* cause for this complex behaviour and this has often been reinforced by professionals e.g. blaming a condition such as ADHD or Asperger's syndrome,[2] or else putting all the blame on parenting practices or stressful life events. Although past IPV is a major influence, it does not *inevitably* cause a particular behaviour and often other children in the same family are not violent. It is also quite common for a child to have a diagnostic label – especially ADHD – and to also have been exposed to IPV. Some practitioners attribute the violent behaviour to the ADHD while minimising or ignoring the IPV. Others see the IPV as all-important and neglect the temperamental differences between children exposed to it. In practice there are *always* multiple causes for any complex behaviour and the view of the intergenerational cycle of abuse as inevitable is dangerous as well as inaccurate (Wilcox 2012).

A sense of entitlement

The first journal article to specifically examine CPV mentioned in passing that the children often had a strong sense of entitlement:

> The abdication of authority by the parent and the symmetrical feeling of physical prowess on the part of the adolescent can result in the adolescent's manifesting a grandiose sense of self along with an enormous sense of entitlement.
>
> (Harbin and Maddin 1979: 1290)

While it seems unfair to say that these parents have 'abdicated' their authority, and symmetrical physical prowess is not of *great* importance in CPV (as shown by girls' violence towards fathers), the idea that these children feel highly entitled goes against the ethos of the parent-blaming literature that dominated during the following decades where the role of entitlement was not discussed. If these children are reacting to parental abuse or excessive control, it is difficult to imagine why they would feel over-entitled. I became aware of the application of the idea of entitlement as a factor in violence and abuse through the work of family therapist Alan Jenkins (1990). He talked of abuse occurring when *Entitlement* outweighed *Responsibility*. Jenkins applied this idea to IPV and to sexual abuse. I found the idea applicable to my work with male perpetrators of IPV and soon realised that it was even more relevant to CPV. When I began exploring these ideas with parents they found it useful and gave countless examples of children's inflated feelings of entitlement. I gradually came to see entitlement as the product of intensive, indulgent parenting interacting with a child's temperament – combined with societal changes which affect all of our children to a greater or lesser extent. I use a visual representation in the form of scales (see Figure 2.1):

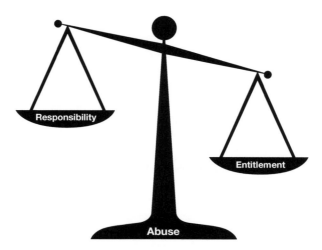

FIGURE 2.1 Responsibility versus Entitlement

This simple formulation appeals to parents and is often helpful to them. It frames the problem as one that they have contributed to – and hence one that they can help alleviate – but in a sympathetic way. They have not been *bad parents*, or cruel, selfish or neglectful, but overall too child-focused. Their children take them for granted because they were always there for them. They have often tried to be their child's friend, but the child sees them not as a friend but as a servant. It is easy to become abusive towards a servant.

In the *Who's in Charge?* group, the concept of entitlement is mainly conveyed through a handout and a brief discussion. It does not require much time or elaborate exercises because parents understand the concept very quickly. The concept not only contributes to an understanding of why some children, and some families, experience CPV (while others do not), but it helps parents understand frequent triggers for violence and helps them work towards reducing entitlement and encouraging responsibility.

Power and responsibility

How can a pre-teen terrorise two parents who tower over him or her? I have seen a petite 12-year-old physically harass a father who dwarfs her and who is clearly far more physically powerful. Why do parents feel helpless and powerless when they objectively control the resources and make most of the decisions in the family's life? What gives these teen terrorists (and pre-teen bullies) their power within the home when their siblings do not appear to wield similar power? In the *Who's in Charge?* group we perform an exercise where parents brainstorm all the ways that parents influence, control or have power over their children. They often need a little prompting about things that are taken for granted, such as parents' decision-making over housing, schools, big family purchases, holidays, food, etc. We have no problem filling a whiteboard with ideas. Next we repeat the exercise with the heading '*How do children influence, control or have power over parents?*' These parents are quick to mention violence, intimidation, threats, destruction of property, disrupting routines and stubborn defiance. In this context they need prompting for the few ways that children can legitimately influence their family (such as suggestions, consultation, persuasion, being lovable). Even with prompting we never fill a whiteboard and the ways that children exert major influence or control – as forms of disruption and abuse – are very evident.

Children in most families are rather powerless. They don't choose if they want to go to school, which school they attend, when is bedtime, and whether to live on ice-cream and chocolate. Most children are quite happy to have their parents guide them: making choices can be stressful when you are impulsive and immature. Yet as responsible caring parents, our actions are dictated by the needs and desires of our children. I would argue that this is increasingly the case with modern, child-focused, *intensive parenting* (Hays 1996). But it is also true that children have little or no 'power' over irresponsible parents. Many more fathers than mothers opt out of parenting, whether physically and/or emotionally, and children exert no power whatsoever over these neglectful parents. The amount of power children have appears to be largely determined by how responsible the parent is. As Crossley (2005) argues:

> power is not held by one party or another but rather consists in the balance or ratio between parties, a ratio which may change over time. To give an example used by Elias, a newly born child, though very much dependent upon its parents and thus subject to their power, can exert considerable influence upon their behaviour, not least because they love it and want it to be happy. To that extent it too has power.
>
> (Crossley 2005: 215)

In intimate relationships a common form of power is when there is a disparity of responsibility. I first became aware of this phenomenon when running groups for separated parents. The women attending the groups thought their ex-partners had a lot of power but the men attending felt powerless. It became clear that responsible fathers (who chose to attend these groups) do not have much power if they are trying hard not to upset their children, but 'access fathers' who are irresponsible about their role, for example by being willing to use the children against their ex-partner, can be very powerful indeed (at least in the short term).

Unrequited love puts one person in a very powerful position and makes the other relatively powerless: disruptive individuals, whether children in class or the loud-mouthed thug in public places, exert temporary power over those who want to act responsibly. Suicide bombers and rogue states exert wildly disproportionate amounts of power in the world. I must stress that the vast majority of these children do love their parents (it is seldom an attachment issue) and they are not generally uncaring (though a few are). Abuse is not about love but about respect and responsibility. They may care deeply about some things and show empathy towards their friends, babies or puppies. The devil is in the detail. It is the fact of not caring about the niceties of everyday life that can give some children power over adults – but only when the adults care about these things. A typical example is a child who has mixed feelings about attending school and does not mind being late. I have known parents spend a frustrating hour or two getting a teenager up for school, giving them a lift because they've missed the bus, and this makes the parent late for work. Other children in the family may be almost as frustrated as the parent as they want to get to school on time and the troublesome child can disrupt and control their schedules. If a neglectful parent doesn't care if the child gets to school, the child has no power in this situation. So an irresponsible parent is less easy to control, and CPV is less likely.

Some children are not embarrassed by making scenes in public and I have heard of a number who will stand on the front lawn screaming abuse for the neighbours to hear. Their parents are humiliated and in a catch-22 situation: if they do nothing they appear weak and pathetic, but if they use force – for example, by dragging the child indoors – then one of the neighbours may report them to child protection services. Seventy-five per cent of the children in my sample destroy property of some kind. Some children target their parents' most prized possessions e.g. flamboyantly smashing family heirlooms or cutting up treasured photos. So the answer to the question 'what gives disruptive, aggressive children power within the family?' is fairly simple but one that we seem to avoid seeing. It has been suggested, and it makes sense to me, that one of the reasons for the common tendency to blame victims is that we try to see the world as a just and fair place, against the ample evidence to the contrary (Lerner 1980). For similar reasons, there is a reluctance to see that being irresponsible provides short-term power – because it's not fair!

Evaluation of the *Who's in Charge?* group program

One of the reasons we have a follow-up session two months after session eight is because it enables a more meaningful evaluation of the impact of the group on changes in the family. Parents complete a questionnaire on the first session with two sets of ratings. The first set of ratings measures general wellbeing and empowerment, and asks parents to rate questions such as 'I feel I can control my child', 'I am feeling stressed or very anxious'. Improvement in these ratings is impressive and even 'My health is suffering' shows a significant positive change. The second set of ratings focuses specifically on their child's behaviour and asks parents how often, in the past two months, their child has hit them, damaged property or been verbally abusive to them, their partner and siblings. Changes in the children's behaviour are less consistent than changes in the parents, as might be expected given that some of these children have been abusive over a number of years. It would not be in keeping with the philosophy of the group to give parents excessively high expectations, but over two-thirds of the young people do show significant changes in reported behaviour. This is particularly encouraging since parents are often more conscious and aware of their child's abusive behaviour after having completed the group: their consciousness-raising about abuse is likely to shape their recognition of it. While this constitutes anecdotal evidence, a formal evaluation has recently been completed, and outcome measures are statistically significant. A published qualitative evaluation also concluded that the *Who's in Charge?* group appeared to meet its objectives (O'Connor 2007).

Notes

1   *Attention deficit hyperactivity disorder* (ADHD) is classed as a neurodevelopmental disorder in DSM-5 and is characterised by a persistent pattern of behaviour that features *inattention* (e.g. easily distracted) and/or *hyperactivity-impulsivity* (e.g. fidgets, interrupts others) (American Psychiatric Association 2013).

2   *Asperger's syndrome* was a developmental disorder characterised by problems in social interaction, communication and flexible thinking, although it does not feature any intellectual impairment. While it constituted a diagnostic category in the previous *Diagnostic and Statistical Manual* (DSM-IV), it has now been subsumed within the broader diagnostic category of *autism spectrum disorders* (ASD) in DSM-5 (APA 2013).

References

American Psychiatric Association. (2013). *Diagnostic and statistical manual of mental disorders* (5th edn.). Washington, DC, Author.

Bonnick, H. (2006). *Access to help for parents feeling victimised or experiencing violence at the hands of their teenage children*. King's College London, University of London. MA in Child Studies.

Brezina, T. (1999). Teenage violence toward parents as an adaptation to family strain. *Youth & Society* 30(4): 416–444.

Browne, K. D. and C. E. Hamilton (1998). Physical violence between young adults and their parents: Associations with a history of child maltreatment. *Journal of Family Violence* 13(1): 59–79.

Caplan, P. J. (1998). Mother-blaming. In. M. Ladd-Taylor and L. Umansky (eds.) *'Bad' mothers: The politics of blame in twentieth-century America*. New York, New York University Press (pp. 127–144)

Caplan, P. J. and I. Hall-McCorquodale (1985). Mother-blaming in major clinical journals. *American Journal of Orthopsychiatry* 55: 345–353.

Cottrell, B. (2004). *When teens abuse their parents*. Halifax, Nova Scotia, Fernwood.

Crossley, N. (2005). *Key concepts in critical theory*. London, Sage.

Eckstein, N. J. (2002). *Adolescent-to-parent abuse: A communicative analysis of conflict processes present in the verbal, physical or emotional abuse of parents*. Lincoln, University of Nebraska (p. 285).

Gallagher, E. (2004a). Parents victimised by their children. *Australian and New Zealand Journal of Family Therapy* 25(1): 1–12.

Gallagher, E. (2004b). Youth who victimise their parents. *Australian and New Zealand Journal of Family Therapy* 25(2): 94–105.

Harbin, H. and D. Maddin (1979). Battered parents: A new syndrome. *American Journal of Psychiatry* 136, 1288–1291.

Harris, J. R. (1998). *The nurture assumption: Why children turn out the way they do*. New York, Free Press.

Hays, S. (1996). *The cultural contradiction of motherhood*. New Haven, CT, Yale University Press.

Holt, A. (2013). *Adolescent-to-parent abuse: Current understandings in policy, practice and research*. Bristol, Policy Press.

Jeffers, S. (1999). *I'm okay, you're a brat*. NSW, Hodder.

Jenkins, A. (1990). *Invitations to responsibility*. Adelaide, Dulwich Centre Publications.

Lerner, M. J. (1980). *The belief in a just world*. New York, Plenum Press.

Mitchell, E. B. (2006). *The violent adolescent: A study of violence transmission across generations*. PhD thesis, University of California, Davis.

O'Connor, R. (2007). *Who's in Charge? A group for parents of violent or beyond control children: Is this group achieving its aims?* Department of Legal Studies; Faculty of Education, Humanities, Law and Theology, Flinders University.

Omer, H. (2000). *Parental presence*. Phoenix, AZ, Zeig, Tucker & Co.

Samenow, S. (1989). *Before it's too late*. New York, Times Books.

Straus, M. A., Gelles, R. J. and Steinmetz., S. K. (1980). *Behind closed doors: Violence in the American family*. Anchor, Doubleday.

Wilcox, P. (2012). Is parent abuse a form of domestic violence? *Social Policy & Society* 11(2), 277–288.

3

HELPING ABUSED PARENTS BY NON-VIOLENT RESISTANCE

Haim Omer

Introduction

In clinical settings, parents are no longer only viewed as helpers in the treatment of their children: they are clients in their own right. After all, a parent's pain is no less real and deserves no less help than a child's pain. This position is most obviously the case in families where parents are abused by their child. Improving the well-being of parents in these families is not only highly justified in itself, but it is also likely to benefit the child, particularly if the improvements are achieved through a method designed to increase parental presence in a non-violent and non-escalating way. This is what parental training in non-violent resistance (NVR) is designed to achieve. NVR was originally developed in the socio-political arena. Groups that were politically disadvantaged and were morally opposed to the use of violence in their fight against exploitation and oppression – but who felt that dialogue and persuasion by themselves were ineffective – developed a variety of non-violent methods for conducting their struggle. The foremost authority in the history, principles and strategies of non-violent resistance is Gene Sharp (1973, 2005), who has described the scope of the approach and its influence in numerous confrontations throughout modern history. NVR as an approach to parent training was developed by a systematic adaptation of the methods described by Sharp to the family arena to help parents deal with aggressive, maladaptive and/or self-destructive behaviors from their children.[1]

The rationale for using non-violent resistance (NVR)

The theoretical and clinical rationale for using NVR with abused parents is linked to a number of factors:

Helplessness

Abused (as well as abusive) parents often view themselves as having less power than the child (Bugental *et al.*, 1989; Bugental *et al.*, 1997) and feel defeated in advance when it comes to withstanding inappropriate demands or standing up to confrontations. Some of these parents vent their frustration by reacting punitively or violently towards their child, others consistently submit to the child's demands, and others oscillate between aggression and submission (Chamberlain & Patterson, 1995). Training in NVR reduces *parental helplessness*, *parental submission* and *parental violence* – the three negative parental reactions that perpetuate the cycle of abuse (Lavi-Levavi, Schachar, & Omer, 2013; Olleffs *et al.*, 2009; Weinblatt & Omer, 2008).

Escalation

The cycle of abuse is fed by the two types of escalation that were described by Bateson (1972): *complementary escalation*, in which parental submission increases the child's demands and abuse, and *reciprocal escalation*, in which hostility begets hostility and abuse multiplies. NVR was specifically designed to counter both kinds of escalation (Omer, 2004).

Power and control

It is not the case that all use of power is illegitimate. Gandhi, the most uncompromising apostle of non-violence, emphasized that demands or entreaties that are not backed by the *power to resist* have little influence (Sharp, 1973, 2005). The language of NVR is thus explicitly a language of struggle. The philosophy of NVR postulates that a person or group that desists on principle from fighting ultimately contributes to the perpetuation of violence. The fight, however, should be a strictly non-violent one. The non-violent resistor must learn to avoid any form of physical or verbal attack and refrain from actions or expressions that aim to humiliate or insult. We therefore talk openly about the parents' *fight* against the child's abusive behaviors, but this 'fight' is profoundly different from what is commonly meant by the word because:

a)   Parents commit themselves to a strictly non-violent and non-humiliating stance
b)   Parents assume responsibility for their own role in the escalation process
c)   The parents' goal is to protect themselves, resist the child's abusive behaviors and – so far as possible – protect the child against his or her own violence (this is in contrast to the more usual kind of 'fight' where one's goal is to defeat the adversary)
d)   Parents maintain and foster the positive elements in the child–parent relationship, while continuing their struggle against the child's violence.

These characteristics may justify us in characterizing parental NVR as a *constructive* rather than a *destructive fight* (Alon & Omer, 2006). In NVR, parents aim to *resist* rather than *control* the child's destructive behaviors. As propounded by Gandhi, a central tenet of NVR is that we cannot determine the opponent's response – only our own. Engaging in NVR with the expectation that the opponent will immediately relinquish violence or oppression is illusory. The effects of NVR manifest themselves first of all on the resisting side, as the resistors overcome helplessness, restore their self-esteem and learn how to mobilize their frustration into productive action. These processes create a new situation in which violence and oppression struggle to survive. The same applies to our approach to parent training: parents learn to resist the child's aggression as they develop endurance, control their own reactions and learn how to counter escalation. Our message to parents is: *You don't have to win, but only to resist.* By becoming able to resist, parents' suffering and humiliation diminish even before the child relinquishes his or her violent behavior. But as the conditions that maintain a child's violence recedes, so does their violence.

Habituation

Anyone observing a family in which the parents suffer from abuse will be struck by the fact that the parents often seem to passively accept flagrant offences and attacks. It is often the outside observer who feels the indignation that the parents seem to lack. This apparently passive acceptance is actually the result of a long process of habituation (Patterson, Dishion, & Bank, 1984). After repeatedly feeling that they are helpless to change the cycle of abuse, parents develop the next best survival technique: learning not to notice it. In order to counter the insidious factor of habituation, parents have to be re-sensitized to the child's abuse. Overcoming habituation and passive acceptance is one of the first goals of NVR in the political arena: the oppressed must be helped to re-experience indignation and hope. Actually the two go hand in hand: the hope of resistance allows the oppressed to feel moral indignation, and vice versa. This double process also characterizes parental training in NVR: parents become re-sensitized so that they can notice the abuse and label it as such, at the same time as they learn to react to it by non-violent resistance.

Presence

NVR is highly relevant for parents because it is the only kind of struggle that is conducted through contact and presence. The strategies of NVR in the socio-political arena work chiefly through the resistors' personal interposition and tenacious presence in ways that obstruct the mechanisms of oppression. Classic examples include Gandhi's struggle against the British salt-monopoly by marching to the sea with thousands of followers in order to mine salt with his own hands; the dismantling of racial discrimination in buses in Alabama by the decided action of a small number of Black resistors, who boarded the buses and sat on seats that were reserved for White people; and the many cases of factory occupation by exploited workers who chained themselves to the machinery, thus evincing their tenacity by committing their very bodies to the process of obstruction. Similarly, parental NVR works through tenacious manifestations of parental presence. Parents learn to come in person to the areas where an adolescent engages in destructive activities and to perform *sit-ins* to protest and resist the child's unacceptable actions. In all of these, the message conveyed by the parents is: *We are your parents. We will not be discarded, ignored, intimidated or paralysed.* NVR rejects authoritarian practices that are based on distance and fear and instead emphasizes *presence* – something that is particularly important in cases of abusive children where the temptation to eschew violence by distancing is particularly strong.

Support, openness and transparency

In contrast to clandestine movements of resistance, NVR rejects secrecy and embraces transparency and publicity. There are many reasons for this choice, as outlined by Sharp (1973, 2005):

1   Openness is the only way to mobilize wide support
2   Publicity influences third parties or even members within the violent camp to take a clear stance against violence and destructiveness
3   Transparency increases resistors' commitment to non-violence, which might waver if the resistance were conducted under the veil of secrecy
4   Secrecy stems from fear and often perpetuates fear.

These processes are highly relevant for abused parents and an NVR approach helps parents to lift the veil of secrecy about their child's behavior, the situation at home and their programme of action. Disclosure allows parents to mobilize the support of friends and relatives, thus rescuing the parents from isolation. Readiness to 'go public' with friends and relatives strengthens the parent's commitment to abide by strict non-violence and non-escalation, and this act of courage tends to boost the parents' morale and determination. Furthermore, the presence of external supporters often has the additional effect of strengthening the child's inner voices that oppose his or her own violent urges. For these reasons, disclosure and the systematic mobilization of support is one of the mainstays of our programme. While many parents require considerable persuasion to go public (even though the publicity is invariably a selective one: the parents decide who should be involved), the great majority of parents accept the need to do so and gain immeasurably from the transition from lonely resistance to supported resistance.

Respect and reconciliation

Leaders like Gandhi and Martin Luther King did not settle for the absence of violence alone: they demanded (from themselves and from their followers) that acts of resistance be accompanied, as far as humanly possible, by real respect for the adversary. This position does not characterize every non-violent resistance movement, and some have claimed that such demands might deter potential followers (Sharp, 1973). However, there is a deep logic to Gandhi's and King's position, stemming from the assumption that the opponent is not made of one cloth. Acts of respect and reconciliation therefore serve to strengthen the positive voices within the violent camp: in contrast, eschewing such acts or engaging in humiliating behaviors would strengthen the violent voices. In the context of parent–child relations, this argument is particularly valid. Our basic assumption is that love still exists between the parents and the abusive child, even if it is sometimes buried under the abuse. Parental acts of respect and reconciliation (that do not include surrender) are thus based on existent feelings, increasing the likelihood that these feelings may feed positive interactions. In our program parents often report that their initiation of acts of reconciliation (e.g. messages of appreciation, symbolic treats, proposing joint activities, acknowledging past offences) strengthens their determination to resist, rather than weakens it. Reconciliation gestures release them from the role of 'the bad guys' and allows them to take steps of resistance without guilt.

Resisting abuse with NVR: practical steps

1. Consciousness-raising

The first step in the program is to help the parents become conscious of the fact that they are victims of abuse and that they can and should resist the abuse in non-violent ways. The process of consciousness-raising regarding i) the fact of abuse, and ii) the possibility of resistance is one and the same. By being made aware of the possibility of non-violent resistance, parents become able to perceive the abuse in ways that do not lead to further escalation and despair. Simply fanning parental indignation against the abuse without offering parents a constructive option of resistance may lead to extreme reactions that would actually reinforce the cycle of coercion. For this reason it is vital to conduct the process of consciousness-raising on a double plane: by raising awareness that violence can be resisted non-violently and by re-sensitizing the parents to situations of abuse. One of the important elements in this process is to highlight to parents how impulsive reactions can feed the coercion cycle and by providing the child with a justification to continue using violence.

2. Anti-escalation training

Child-to-parent abuse does not usually arise out of nothing: it is often preceded by an emotional crescendo that is unwittingly fanned by the parents' own reactions. During the therapy sessions, situations of escalation are examined and reactions that express self-control are formulated and rehearsed (Omer, 2004;

Case study: Jerry

Jerry (12 years old) was socially well adjusted, well liked at the boy scouts and in his soccer team, and was an average student at school. However, at home his behavior was markedly different: he was extremely demanding and offensive towards his mother, using violent threats and actions towards her, and would ignore his father who, on a few occasions, had reacted to his abusive behavior by slapping him. Now when his father tried to intervene during Jerry's abusive interactions with his mother, Jerry would shut him up provocatively ('Did anybody talk to you?' 'Was your opinion asked by anyone?') and would threaten to call the police if his father touched him. Ever since his father reacted to his abuse by slapping him, Jerry carried a lancet with him, which he had received as a gift from a friend who was the son of a surgeon. Jerry had shown the lancet to his mother on occasion, as a threat to underscore his demands. A detailed interview with Jerry's parents did not reveal any history of violence from Jerry's father towards Jerry or any other family member, until the events in the last year when Jerry's father felt he had been 'forced to react as he did'. Jerry's father felt that his son's violence, and his ostracism of him, had divested him of his fatherhood: he felt increasingly marginalized and helpless. Raising the parents' awareness that Jerry's abusive behavior was maintained both by the mother's submission and the father's oscillation between enforced passivity and impulsive reactions was the first treatment goal. This process was carried out hand-in-hand with an introduction to NVR. Jerry's actions were labelled as 'abuse' and 'violence' and his parents were asked to write down a detailed list of Jerry's actions towards them or his siblings that typified the abuse. As is often the case in this re-sensitization phase, the parents were surprised in their discovery of how frequent and painful the abusive interactions were, not only for themselves but for their other children.

Weinblatt & Omer, 2008). We have coined three phrases that illustrate the non-escalating stance of NVR, which parents should keep in mind:

> Strike the iron, when it is cold!
> You can't control the child, but only yourselves!
> You don't have to win, but only to persist!

Each of these phrases carries a special meaning in the abusive situation. The first expression (*Strike the iron, when it is cold!*) is designed to help parents overcome the urge to react immediately to the child's unacceptable behaviors. The rationale is that immediate reactions come about at the height of arousal and increase the risk of escalation. Any wish, demand or problem that may have given rise to the abusive interaction is now defined as one that should be given attention only 'when the iron is cold'. Parents learn to take a deep breath, postpone the temptation for immediate action and develop planned ways to resist the abuse and the inappropriate demands that are linked to it. Parents do not stay passive at the moment of the abuse, but react in ways that signal their new attitude. For example, a verbally abused parent may say to their child: 'I won't react now to what you are saying, but I will consider how best to protect myself and will get back to this issue later.' The child may react derisively, but the parent knows that they mean it. After one or two instances in which the parent comes up with a prepared and delayed response, the child understands that the parent is no longer a passive victim. In more urgent cases, when the child stages a physical attack, the parent should eschew the attack and start contacting supporters. In a number of cases the attacked parent (usually the mother of a highly violent adolescent) has enclosed herself in the bedroom or water closet and called a number of supporters by telephone. Preparing the supporters beforehand for such an eventuality turns the negative crisis into a manifestation of resistance.

The second expression (*You can't control the child, but only yourselves!*) aims to modify dominant attitudes (such as 'I am the boss!') that often turn the parent–child relationship into a zero-sum game (Bugental, Lyon, & Cortez, 1997). The shift from attempting to control the other to exercising self-control is a key element of the skill-set learned in NVR parental training (Lavi-Levavi, Schahar, & Omer, 2013; Omer, 2004; Weinblatt & Omer, 2008). Parents learn to say explicitly: 'I can't control your mouth (or your hands), but I can control myself.' Emphasizing self-control rather than control over a child changes a central aspect in the escalation of abusive interactions: the attempt to stop a verbally abusive child by yelling at him or her: 'You will shut your mouth!' is usually an invitation for the child to prove the parent wrong. In NVR, the compulsion to control is replaced by a duty to resist. In resisting, we know full well that we have no control over the other, but the positive strength conveyed by resistance more than outweighs the parents' candid acknowledgment that they have no ultimate control over the child.

The third expression (*You don't have to win, but only to persist!*) is actually a synthesis of the other two expressions: it unites the factor of time with the renunciation of control. The message of persistence is a good antidote to the sense of total urgency that exacerbates an abusive interaction. In treatment, the parents are helped to develop a time-span that arches over days, weeks and months, instead of minutes. This not only enables parents to protect themselves, but it also offers the child an anchor which they may gradually become able to utilize, so as to stabilize him- or herself (Omer *et al.*, 2013). In an escalating interaction, a child's impulsive urge is multiplied by that of their parents. We have described elsewhere a similar situation where the anxiety of the child is multiplied by the parents' anxiety that the child might panic (Lebowitz & Omer, 2013). In our treatment for parents of abusive (as well as of anxious) children, we help parents to counter this by conveying a new message: 'We thought we could not withstand your abuse (or anxiety). We are now able to do so, and we are sure that you can also withstand your urge.'

3. The announcement

During the first few sessions, parents are helped to prepare a semi-formal 'announcement', in which they declare to their child that they will resist the abuse and will no longer keep it secret. The announcement fulfils a number of goals:

1 It serves as an opening event, almost a rite of transition, to a new phase in the family's life
2 It openly states the parents' intentions, thus conferring legitimacy to their actions
3 It introduces the parents to a new kind of interaction, in which they state their position in a self-controlled manner and in a way that is independent of the child's agreement
4 It tells the child that the parents will no longer keep the problem secret
5 It presents a united front to the child (in cases where this is possible, the parents should deliver the announcement jointly. Single parents may be helped to deliver the announcement by having a supporter present at the time of delivery).

The parents deliver the announcement verbally and in written form, usually in the child's room. Here is a typical example:

> Dear Tom
>
> We will no longer accept any abusive behaviors from you. We will no longer be passive, but will resist threats, physical violence and curses to the best of our abilities and by any possible means, except hitting you back. We will not stay alone but will get help from anybody that is willing to help us. We have understood that violence is not a private event and this justifies us in getting this help. We do this because we are not willing to lose you or to let the violence poison our lives.
>
> Your loving parents.

With the therapist's help, parents rehearse how to deliver the announcement and how to develop non-escalating responses to their child's reactions. Parents often say: 'She will never agree', 'He will tear it apart', 'He will run away'. This is a good opportunity to make it clear that NVR does not depend on the child's agreement. Thus, if the child refuses to listen or read, the parents leave the announcement on the table. If the child tears the page, parents can say: 'We didn't expect you to agree. We are giving you this to be fair with you, so that you may know what we are going to do.' When parents succeed in delivering the announcement in this spirit (and the majority are able do so), they are already on the way to becoming non-violent resistors.

4. The support group

Whenever possible, we conduct a supporters' meeting. In preparation for that meeting, parents are helped to write a message for the supporters, giving a brief description of the problem and asking for their help. The following is a typical example:

> Dear Silvia and Jack
>
> As you now know, Mary has been very abusive and violent towards us, and especially towards Silvia. We are now in a parent-therapy, in which we are learning to resist Mary's violence in determined but strictly non-violent ways. We now understand that in remaining alone and keeping the problem secret we were making it worse. So we would like to invite you to a supporters' meeting together with our therapist. We would also be very glad if you could visit us at home sometime during the next few weeks and, if Mary agrees, have a short conversation with her. If she doesn't agree, you could leave her a short written message. In any case, your visit will be enormously important to us.
>
> Your friends Albert and Jenny

Many parents have trouble going public, because they feel ashamed, because they fear this might be detrimental to their child, or because it may produce a violent reaction from their child. Dealing with these objections is one of the central tasks and skills of the NVR therapist. The recruitment of other parents who have previously undergone the treatment can be of great help in convincing parents who are new to the program. In cases where a supporters' meeting does not materialize, supporters can be recruited on an individual basis. Typical supporters include grandparents and other members of the extended family, friends of the parents and sometimes the parents of the child's friends. The supporters do not have to live nearby because their help can be made available by phone or email. We have often made use of supporters who lived abroad, especially with migrant families: help from grandparents or other members of the extended family who call from abroad to talk with the abusive child can be very effective.

Resistance steps

The majority of resistance steps can be subsumed under three categories: a) Documentation and involvement of supporters b) Sit-ins, and c) Planned withdrawal of services.

a) Documentation and involvement of supporters

The very fact that supporters are informed of the abuse and that it is made clear to the child that they have been notified and will do all in their power to help, constitutes a significant act of resistance. No child or adolescent is immune from public opinion, although many may try to put up a show of indifference. The best way for parents to proceed is to start documenting the abuse – in writing or by visual means – when the child behaves abusively. We do not recommend that the parents record the abuse as it is occurring as this often leads to escalation. Writing and photographing are better because they can be conducted *when the iron is cold*. The documentation is then sent to the supporters, who later call the child. It is not necessary that all supporters call the child: one or two each time is enough. However, it is important that parents tell their child that they are no longer keeping the events secret and that they will send their reports to whomever they feel is appropriate. Supporters are specifically asked to address the child in a positive way, but to make clear that they know what happened, that they view the behavior as violent and unacceptable, and that they believe that the child can overcome the violence. Here follows a typical phone call by a grandfather from abroad:

> Hello Mark. This is grandpa speaking! Your mother called me this afternoon. I was surprised because I knew it was very late at night in Tel-Aviv, as the time difference from here is six hours. She told me about the fight you had and the names that you called her. She also told me that you threw down your plate with the food on the floor. You know that I love you and am eagerly expecting your visit in the summer. But this has to stop. It is violence and it is abuse. If you are angry with your ma, you can call me and I will help you calm down. But you simply cannot go on like this. I trust you and I am sure you can deal with those incidents in a better way . . . Yes, I understand that you have complaints, and I am willing to help you to find a reasonable solution. But hitting around or cursing will not be part of any such solution. I'll be in touch with you and will ask your ma to update me on a daily basis.

In therapy, considerable attention is given to prepare parents for dealing with the child's reactions. This preparation strengthens the parents enormously. After involving supporters in a planned manner and being able to withstand the backlash, the parents are changed. There is probably no single intervention in the whole NVR repertory that has such a profound influence on the parents and on the abusive interaction.

b) The sit-in

The sit-in has come to typify NVR in families, probably because it is emblematic of NVR in the socio-political arena. It is important to understand that the sit-in is a measure of resistance and not a disciplinary step geared to changing the child's immediate behavior. In fact, the sit-in affects the parents more than the child: in preparing for the sit-in, creating possible scripts for its development and staging it in a self-controlled manner, the parents achieve a high proficiency in NVR.

A case study

An obese single mother of a violent 15-year-old girl staged a sit-in after the daughter had kicked her and stolen her money. She was supported over the phone by her brother, whom the daughter respected. The mother sat on a chair that blocked the door. The daughter, who otherwise would have attacked her, refrained from doing so because her uncle was listening. Instead, she tried to silently push her mother, but her mother stuck to her ground. After a few minutes, the daughter gave up, whispered a few curses and lay down on the bed with her face to the wall. The mother remained in the room for a whole hour, in complete silence. During the next therapy session, the mother reported the sit-in experience and suddenly started to grin. The therapist asked her about it, and the mother said: 'It was the first time in my life that I didn't regret not to have gone on a diet!' The experience of this sit-in became emblematic for the mother's new 'sense of weight'. Although there was no proposal and the daughter maintained an appearance of non-cooperation, the mother's feeling and standing were profoundly affected.

Thus, the sit-in can be viewed as training in a real-life context. In the sit-in, the parents come into the child's room (a single parent may be accompanied by a supporter, in person or via technology), sit down and tell the child: 'We are here because we are no longer willing to accept the kind of abusive behavior that you displayed today. We will sit here and wait for a proposal as to how the abuse might end.' After this opening, the parents stay silent, as best and for as long as they can. In preparation, the therapist can help the parents to develop ways of coping with typical reactions to the sit-in, such as physical attacks and attempts to expel them, ignore them or deride them (Omer, 2004, 2011). The sit-in usually takes between 30 minutes and one hour. If the child makes a proposal, a dialogue may ensue. If not, the parents are advised not to raise proposals of their own. The success of the sit-in is not a function of the proposals, but of the readiness of the parents to sit through it. After the sit-in has been performed, the therapist goes over the parents' report in detail, stressing the positive elements and focusing on their experience of having manifested *presence* in a determined way. This often produces a new kind of self-awareness, in which parents become more conscious of their own strength and are less 'hypnotized' by the child's negative reactions.

c) Planned withdrawal of services

Although the temporary withdrawal of services from the aggressive child may share a resemblance with 'usual punishments', the spirit in which it is conducted in NVR is very different. Services are not withdrawn as a negative reinforcement, so as to shape the child's behavior. Indeed, parents are specifically told that their child may refuse to improve his or her behavior in order to save face and avoid feeling like they are on the losing side. The withdrawal of services in NVR tells the child (and the parents!) that, in a context of violence, services that are otherwise willingly and lovingly given become tokens of exploitation. By refusing services temporarily, the parents say: 'We won't be passive victims of exploitation.' If a supporter echoes this message, it makes an even greater impact. For example, in one case a teen-driver was abusive to his parents and was told by a supporter: 'I know your parents stopped giving you the car for a week. They did this because they felt, rightfully, that you had humiliated your mother. If you don't show respect to your mother, your parents will restore their own self-worth by refusing to be exploited.' The supporter may then propose to help in the negotiation of an acceptable solution for both sides. Even if the proposal is not taken up by the child, the message does not lose its impact.

The withdrawal of services works best when it is temporary and when it does not damage otherwise positive interactions with the child. The withdrawal is not accompanied by a refusal to speak with the child, as such refusal would lead to a deepening of the mutual distancing. Neither is it accompanied by conditional clauses like 'You won't get the car until you start to behave respectfully' because such a condition would deepen the tug-of-war. Withdrawal of services is actually a symbolic act of protest, by which the parents overcome their passive victimhood in a way that is legitimized by the surroundings (i.e. the supporters). Like the sit-in, it is part and parcel of the process of resistance and not a single measure that brings about compliance. When parents reinstate the service, they may tell the child: 'We are giving this back to you because we love you.' This message can be reinforced by a supporter, who may say to the child: 'I talked to your mother. She no longer feels deeply offended, so she feels she can give you back the car with a good feeling.' There is no need to get the child to agree – it is enough if the message is relayed. In this way, the restitution of withdrawn services is a spontaneous gesture of reconciliation. Such gestures are very important in NVR.

5. Reconciliation gestures

Even when parents are tenaciously resisting violence and humiliation, they are encouraged to make loving and appreciative gestures to the child. These gestures are not a prize for good behavior, but are unconditional manifestations of care. Their value, however, is far more than sentimental: they are designed to reinstitute the parents as independent agents and to strengthen the positive voices within the child. They are thus an integral part of the process of resistance.

Parents often object when the idea of free reconciliation gestures is proposed: 'She will think we are weak!' This remark offers an opportunity for a discussion about positive strength. The position in NVR is that parental strength is not conditional on the child's acknowledgment, but on the parents' own actions, their own support network and on their willingness to persevere in ways they feel are

---

Case study: Shawn

Shawn (12 years old) developed a hit-and-run style of behaving towards his mother: he would scream offences at her and lock himself in his room, playing computer games for hours. His mother had already canvassed the help of a couple of friends and a neighbour and had performed a sit-in. Shawn had reacted by locking himself away for even longer hours. Shawn's mother knocked at his door and said: 'I have baked a cheesecake for you.' Shawn screamed: 'I don't want any cake from you!' His mother replied: 'OK, I made it because I know how much you like it. But I can't force you to eat it. I'll put it in the fridge.' She then went away without another word. Shawn felt he was honour-bound to ignore his mother's offer and not even taste the cake. The next day his mother threw away the cake. A few days later, she knocked at his door and the initial scene repeated itself. However, this time Shawn felt that his self-respect had been safeguarded by his first vocal refusal and not eating the cake again was simply too much. So, when his mother was not present, he went to the fridge and ate from the cake. In parallel, Shawn's offensive behavior, as well as the time he spent enclosed in his room, gradually diminished. We believe that a piece of his mother's cake in the child's stomach enabled some positive reconciliatory work. From his mother's side, offering the cake but going away and leaving Shawn to his own simmering frustration allowed her to feel that she was both a good mother and a strong mother. Part of her renewed strength came from the fact that her love was no longer dependent on Shawn's reactions. The game of mutual refusal had been broken, and Shawn's mother also felt that she knew better how to protect herself.

---

right, instead of in response to their child's moods. In the case study above, the parent had planned in advance how she would react to her child's refusal. She knew she would not continue distressing discussions with him, or repeatedly ask him to open the door, or blame him for refusing her love. By expecting his refusal and telling him 'I can't force you to eat it. I did it because I love you' and then silently walking away, she regained a sense of agency. Her son was left with his offences stuck in his own throat – and with a watering, if angry, mouth. In a couple of weeks, the positive gestures added their positive weight to the resistance measures, allowing for a new cycle to develop.

The most common reconciliation steps are messages of appreciation, symbolic gifts, proposals of pleasurable joint activities, offers of small unrequested services, reminders of *positive* events from the past, and the expression of regret for past parental mistakes (Omer, 2004). Jakob *et al.* (2014) have argued that such gestures, when performed in the context of NVR, are often able to renew the 'dialogue of care' that had previously been obstructed by the hardships of parenting a difficult and aggressive child.

Applications and clinical considerations – how and when to tread carefully

Parental training in NVR has been implemented with abused parents or carers of children from a range of age groups and who exhibit a range of clinical conditions, when the child is living at home or in an institutional setting. Examples include children of school age with externalizing disorders (Omer, 2004; Weinblatt & Omer, 2008), children diagnosed with obsessive-compulsive disorder (OCD) and other anxiety disorders (Lebowitz et al., 2013), children in foster families (van Holen, 2014), hospitalized psychotic adolescents (Goddard et al., 2009), adult children with 'entitled dependency' (Lebowitz et al., 2012), and adult children diagnosed with Asperger's syndrome (Shiloh, Golan & Omer, in press). Although these groups may be very diverse, the abusive interactions tend to be quite similar. NVR training is also helpful for parents of abusive children who do not fit any diagnostic label. However, while we have not identified any diagnostic counter-indications, there are a number of peculiarities and danger zones that should be given careful consideration.

A common concern of both parents and professionals is the fear that the child might direct the violence against themselves, perhaps in response to the parents' resistance measures. Many children or adolescents who are violent against their parents also threaten suicide, and such threats should never be lightly dismissed. However, in many cases the threat of suicide is also a clear aggressive act against the parents. This is apparent when the threat is raised to support a demand for services, or as an attempt to get the parents off the child's back, or in the context of blaming the parents for past and present faults. The parents' reaction to the threat is a crucial factor that may affect suicidal risk. In addition, parents suffer greatly under such threats and their suffering deserves support just as much as the child's suffering and we have developed a detailed program to help parents cope with suicide threats (Omer & Dolberger, in press). The justification for implementing NVR in those situations is that it allows parents to resist the threat while at the same time lending support to the suicidal child. NVR enables parents to cope with the threat in its acute phase (the *containment stage* of the intervention) while also increasing their ability to deal constructively with the interactional patterns that are connected to the threat (the *anchoring stage* of the intervention). We would advise professionals who are dealing with children, adolescents or young adults who are both aggressive and suicidal to acquaint themselves with our approach to suicide threats.

Other clinical conditions may require an adaptation of the present approach. For example, violence towards parents can be a common feature of obsessive-compulsive disorder[2] (OCD) (Lebowitz et al., 2011) and other anxiety disorders, with violence erupting when parents attempt to reduce their accommodation to the child's anxiety. In fact, reducing parental accommodation is essential when treating anxiety disorders in children, as high parental accommodation has been shown to be a strong predictor of negative outcomes (Merlo et al., 2009).

The difficulty here mirrors that of the parents of the suicidal child: how can the parents resist and support at the same time? Again, NVR offers a good response to this dilemma: our program for parents of anxious children deals with both aspects of the problem in parallel (Lebowitz & Omer, 2013). A systematic study of ten families where children refused any therapy showed that an NVR-based program succeeded in improving child symptomatology, reducing aggression against the parents and increasing the likelihood of the child becoming willing to participate in individual therapy, so as better to cope with the anxiety on his or her own (Lebowitz *et al.*, 2013).

Another adaptation of NVR involves the parents of adolescents and young adults with Asperger's syndrome.[3] Such children can become aggressive, especially when their strict demands for 'ideal' surroundings are not met. In this case, we modified our procedure in ways that addressed the special needs of these young people, especially regarding their difficulties in mentalization. Parents are helped to use the delay period in their reactions (*Strike the iron, when it is cold!*) and to formulate messages that help stimulate mentalization. For example, a young man with Asperger's syndrome, who had aggressive bouts whenever his father required help with the laundry, was regularly given messages like: 'You are not doing your part. I guess you are attacking me because you feel over-burdened, yet your screaming hurts me and makes me feel very frustrated. If you need me to explain again how the rotation works, or how to work the washing machine, I will be happy to do that. Yet, if this reoccurs, I will understand you don't want to take part in the rotation of duties, therefore each of us will be responsible for his own clothes' (Shiloh, Golan, & Omer, submitted).

This brings us to the special issue of violence against parents perpetrated by adult children. This kind of violence is common in the context of what we have termed *entitled dependence* – that is, adult children who remain largely dependent on their parents, often continue living in the parental home and evolve patterns of relating that are damaging for both the parents and for themselves (Lebowitz *et al.*, 2012). Helping those parents face up to the violence involves changing patterns of relating that are deeply ingrained. The violence of adult children can be more frightening than that of a child or adolescent, especially if threats of suicide are involved. Treating these cases requires special preparation by the therapeutic team. In effect, we believe a team is obligatory, even though the therapy is normally conducted by a single therapist. Team-work is required because an isolated therapist will risk feeling overwhelmed by the demands of such cases. Optimally the team would include not only a supportive therapist peer-group, but also a psychiatrist, who can be available for direct work with the adult child (when possible) and for discussing the case with the parents and the therapist. In our experience, interventions with parents of adult children also take longer. While the usual length of treatment for parents of violent children and adolescents ranges between 10 and 12 sessions, treatment with the parents of adults is typically between 15 and 25 sessions. This is because it takes more preparation and more support to get the parents to act. However, despite such difficulties, NVR has been shown to be a highly promising approach to these cases, which are becoming more and more frequent as the proportion of young adults living in their parents' homes steadily grows throughout the industrialized world.

Notes

1   Such behaviors might include truancy, stealing, lying, violence, substance abuse, blackmailing, computer addiction.
2   *Obsessive-compulsive disorder* (OCD) is broadly classed as an anxiety disorder in DSM-5 and is characterized by intrusive thoughts (obsessions) and repetitive behaviors (compulsions) to an extent that interferes with daily life (American Psychiatric Association, 2013)
3   *Asperger's syndrome* was a developmental disorder characterized by problems in social interaction, communication and flexible thinking, although it does not feature any intellectual impairment. While it constituted a diagnostic category in the previous *Diagnostic and Statistical Manual* (DSM-IV), it has now been subsumed within the broader diagnostic category of *autism spectrum disorders* (ASD) in DSM-5 (APA, 2013).

References

Alon, N. & Omer, H. (2006). *The psychology of demonization*. Mahwah, NJ: Lawrence Erlbaum Associates.

American Psychiatric Association. (2013). *Diagnostic and statistical manual of mental disorders* (5th edn.). Washington, DC: Author.

Bateson, G. (1972). *Steps to an ecology of mind*. New York: Ballantine.

Bugental, D. B., Blue, J. B. & Cruzcosa, M. (1989). Perceived control over caregiving outcomes: Implications for child abuse. *Developmental Psychology, 25*, 532–539.

Bugental, D. B., Lyon, J. E., Krantz, J. & Cortez, V. (1997). Who's the boss? Accessibility of dominance ideation among individuals with low perceptions of interpersonal power. *Journal of Personality and Social Psychology, 72*, 1297–1309.

Chamberlain, P. & Patterson, G. R. (1995). Discipline and child compliance in parenting. In M. H. Bornstein (ed.) *Handbook of parenting (Vol. 1)* (pp. 205–225). Mahwah, NJ: Lawrence Erlbaum Associates.

Goddard, N., Van Gink, K., Van der Stegen, B., Van Driel, J. & Cohen, A. P. (2009). 'Smeed het ijzer als het koud is'. Non-violent resistance op een acuut psychiatrische afdeling voor adolescenten. *Maandblad Geestelijke Volksgezondheid, 64*, 531–539.

Golan, O., Shiloh, H. & Omer, H. (in press). Non-violent resistance for the parents of young adults with High Functioning Autism Spectrum Disorders. *Journal of Family Therapy*.

Jakob, P., Wilson, J. & Newman, M. (2014). Nonviolence and a focus on the child: A UK perspective. *Context, 132*, 37–41.

Lebowitz, E. R., Dolberger, D., Nortov, E. & Omer, H. (2012). Parent training in nonviolent resistance for adult entitled dependence. *Family Process, 51*, 90–106.

Lebowitz, E. R. & Omer, H. (2013). *Treating childhood and adolescent anxiety: A guide for caregivers*. Hoboken, NJ: Wiley.

Lebowitz, E. R., Omer, H., Hermes, H. & Scahill, L. (2013). Parent training for childhood anxiety disorders: The SPACE program. *Cognitive and Behavioral Practice, 21*, 456–469.

Lebowitz, E. R., Vitulano, L. A. & Omer, H. (2011). Coercive and disruptive behaviors in pediatric obsessive compulsive disorder. *Psychiatry, 74*, 362–371.

Lavi-Levavi, I., Shachar, I. & Omer, H. (2013). Non-violent resistance and parent–child escalation: The special plight of mothers. *Journal of Systemic Therapies, 32*(4), 79–93.

Merlo, L., Lehmkuhl, H., Geffken, G. & Storch, E. (2009). Decreased family accommodation associated with improved therapy outcome in pediatric obsessive-compulsive disorder. *Journal of Consulting and Clinical Psychology, 77,* 355–360.

Ollefs, B., von Schlippe, A., Omer, H. & Kritz, J. (2009). Youngsters with externalizing behavior problems: Effects of parent-training (in German). *Familiendynamik, 34,* 256–265.

Omer. H. (2004). *Non-violent resistance: A new approach to violent and self-destructive children.* New York: Cambridge University Press.

Omer, H. (2011). *The new authority: Family, school, community.* New York: Cambridge University Press.

Omer, H. & Dolberger, D. I. (in press). Helping parents cope with suicide threats: An approach based on non-violent resistance (NVR). *Family Process.*

Omer, H., Steinmetz, S. G., Carthy, T. & von Schlippe, A. (2013). The anchoring function: Parental authority and the parent–child bond. *Family Process, 52,* 193–206.

Patterson, G. R., Dishion, T. J. & Bank, L. (1984). Family interaction: A process model of deviancy training. *Aggressive Behavior, 10,* 253–267.

Sharp, G. (1973). *The politics of nonviolent action.* Boston, MA: Extending Horizons Books.

Sharp, G. (2005). *Waging nonviolent struggle.* Boston, MA: Extending Horizons Books.

Shiloh, H., Golan, O. & Omer, H. (submitted). Alleviating the 'dependence trap' of young adults with autism spectrum disorders and their parents, through non-violent resistance.

Van Holen, F. (2014). Development and implementation of a training program for foster parents based on nonviolent resistance. Unpublished doctoral dissertation, Vrije Universiteit Brussel, Brussels.

Weinblatt, U. & Omer, H. (2008) Non-violent resistance: A treatment for parents of children with acute behavior problems. *Journal of Marital and Family Therapy, 34,* 75–92.

4

TRAUMA-BASED APPROACHES TO ADOLESCENT-TO-PARENT ABUSE

Jane Evans

Introduction

It is sometimes said that we cannot keep using traumas from the past as an 'excuse' for violence or abuse exhibited in the present. Indeed, the appetite in the adolescent-to-parent abuse world for young people to 'take responsibility' for their actions, albeit in a reparative and restorative way, is a familiar and commonsensical framework for most of us to operate within. However, while I do not condone any kind of abusive or harmful behaviour towards another, when actions are such a transgression against the seemingly 'natural' child–parent relationship I believe we need to fully and deeply understand *why*, rather than merely attempt to 'fix it'. A young person who regularly hits, kicks, bites or threatens their parent, who kicks in doors and punches holes in walls, is acting against their own interests in terms of their basic long-term survival and well-being because it puts them at odds with the person(s) they most rely on for this. Therefore, until we look at adolescent-to-parent abuse within the context of the lived experience of trauma, the role of attachment and the child's relationship with his/her birth parent(s), adolescent-to-parent abuse will continue to make little sense. This chapter traces my journey of making sense of this world and finding ways to work within it.

The 11–17 project at Wish for a Brighter Future

For the past 20 years I have been working with parents, carers, children, young people and families who have complex needs rooted in early childhood trauma. My previous professional roles include working in a pre-school for children with physical and learning disabilities, working in early education, working in an NSPCC[1] Family Centre, working as a social work assistant in a child protection team and working as a parenting worker for a domestic abuse organisation. My experience of direct work with families has informed my understanding of their lived experiences and how this relates to current research and findings around trauma and relational needs. However, for the first nine years of doing this work I did not fully understand what I was dealing with, or have a conceptual framework for understanding it. Fortunately, when being assessed to become a Local Authority respite foster carer with my husband, we were allocated an amazing social worker who looked me in the eye and firmly suggested that I read everything I could on trauma, attachment and brain development. I did, and my practice now integrates research from the fields of neuroscience, neurobiology, attachment and trauma with what families have taught me directly.

My work in the field of adolescent-to-parent abuse began in January 2014 when working as an adolescent and parent relationship worker for a small voluntary organisation called Wish for a Brighter Future in Hartcliffe, Bristol (UK). Wish for a Brighter Future was established in 2003 and had originally been a community-based organisation for victims of domestic abuse. However, changes in funding in 2011 resulted in the organisation shifting their focus to work with teenagers who use, and are impacted by, violence and abuse – both in the home and within their intimate relationships. The post at Wish was funded to work with young people and their parents across the city of Bristol, although many of the referrals were confined to particular areas of economic and social deprivation. Referrals were initially for young people, aged 11–24 years, experiencing and/or using violence and abuse in intimate and/or family relationships. However, with limited funds and only one worker it soon became evident that there needed to be a clear focus on the overwhelming demand for support around adolescent-to-parent abuse, as evidenced in the referrals received. Initial referrals are taken over the phone and although there have been some self-referrals by parents, most have come from professionals, especially via schools and children's services. Work is not undertaken unless the young person is aware of the referral and is willing to engage with the work.

After 12 months of working at Wish I had engaged with approximately 10 young people and 10 parents,[2] some of which involved 'whole family' support. Of these families:

- 9 were single parent families + 8 were families headed by mothers
- 1 family had a step-parent
- 1 young person lived with their father
- 8 White British young people + 2 dual-heritage British young people
- 9 White British parents + 1 African-Caribbean parent
- 6 families had household income derived solely from state benefit payments
- 9 young people had school or college attendance/engagement/exclusion issues
- 1 young person was in part-time employment
- *All* the parents had experience of living with domestic violence and abuse
- *All* the young people had childhood experiences of living with domestic violence and abuse
- *All* the young people had siblings.

The impact of trauma on behaviour and well-being

What I learned from these families was similar to what I have learned from all the families I have ever had the privilege to work with: I did not find anything 'new' or startling in my work with adolescent-to-parent abuse. I went with a genuine curiosity as to what might lie behind a young person being abusive towards their birth parent[3] but I also took a hypothesis with me: that such behaviour is likely to be rooted in trauma and attachment issues from early childhood experiences of domestic abuse and violence, perhaps combined with parental mental and physical illness, substance dependence and other parental difficulties which would impact on a parent's ability to be emotionally available to, and connected with, their developing child.

The impact of trauma can begin before birth: the pre-birth developing brain and body can be impacted by exposure to high levels of stress hormones which can provide the foundations of developmental trauma. In his proposal for a new diagnosis of *developmental trauma disorder* to the American Psychiatric Association, Bessel van der Kolk suggested that 'studies on the sequelae of childhood trauma in the context of caregiver abuse or neglect consistently demonstrate chronic and severe problems with emotional regulation, impulse control, attention and cognition, dissociation, interpersonal relationships, and self and relational schemas' (2014: 158–159). This is an accurate summation of what I have repeatedly seen and heard in families during the course of my professional life, including in families struggling with adolescent-to-parent abuse. I continually meet parents living with their own, often unidentified, childhood trauma who are doing their best to parent children through the haze and maze of its effects. This is often during, or after, an adult abusive relationship(s) which has triggered and exacerbated their earliest traumatic experiences. Unfortunately, parents are all too often presumed to lack 'boundaries' and when children fall outside of acceptable social norms, *permissiveness* becomes a readily available explanation. However, as Routt and Anderson found: 'after interviewing hundreds of abused parents and working with them for months at a time, the permissive parent jacket doesn't fit abused parents' (2015: 62).

Attempting to develop a deeper understanding of how trauma affects all areas of development has been a revelation. One particularly insightful study is the *Adverse Childhood Experiences Study* (the ACE Study) conducted by Felitti and Anda (see Centers for Disease Control and Prevention, 2014). This research was carried out at Kaiser Permanente's Department of Preventative Medicine in San Diego, USA, and the researchers spent more than a year developing ten questions covering carefully defined categories of adverse childhood experiences, including physical and sexual abuse, physical and emotional neglect, and family dysfunction (such as having had parents who were divorced, mentally ill, addicted or in prison). Drawing on data from with 17,421 respondents, the ACE Study produced robust evidence into the commonality of adverse experiences in childhood and how they can impact all areas of adult life. They found that traumatic life experiences during childhood and adolescence are far more common than expected, with 64 per cent of their sample having experienced at least one adverse experience in childhood (Anda *et al.*, 2006). Thirty-eight per cent of the sample experienced multiple adverse experiences and the researchers found that this produced a cumulative and damaging effect on a variety of behavioural health and social problems, including affective disturbances, poor health outcomes (including substance dependency), poor childhood memory, perceived high stress and increased risks of perpetrating IPV in adulthood (Anda *et al.*, 2006).

The impact of trauma on family life

Many of my professional observations over the years, especially during my work with adolescent-to-parent abuse, resonate with the findings from the ACE study. What follows is a discussion of some of these common themes, discussed in the context of my own work with families where adolescent-to-parent abuse was impacting on the child–parent relationship and causing harm and suffering. My aim is to illustrate the complex needs of families who have lived with repetitive trauma, where daily life rarely feels straightforward for their already-stressed systems and where trauma is repeatedly played out in the over-reaction to apparently low-level occurrences such as running out of bread, an unexpected bill or a 'look' from someone in the corridor at school. Traumatised parents and children have an in-built survival system premised on a perception of life as threatening, unpredictable and potentially traumatic. This raises anxiety and stress levels, making confrontation and conflict more likely.

Mental and physical health

In terms of mental health, I have found that parents and young people have complex needs which often present as depression, chronic anxiety, obsessive compulsive disorder (OCD), attention deficit hyperactivity disorder (ADHD), learning difficulties, self-regulation difficulties, high stress levels and sensory impairment needs. Most of the parents have been prescribed anti-depressants and many make their own decisions as to when to stop and start taking them, in an attempt to self-medicate in the absence of 'trauma-informed' support. The young people had often been referred to Child and Adolescent Mental Health Services (CAMHS) while I was working with them: some received a service, some did not. Young people were suspected of 'having' ADHD, oppositional defiance disorder (ODD), autistic spectrum disorder (ASD) or some other mental disorder.

Physical health can also be compromised by early childhood trauma, something which is well documented in the ACE study. Its ongoing follow-up component has correlated negative health outcomes such as hospitalisation, prescription drug use and premature mortality with adverse childhood experiences (Anda *et al.*, 2010). Unfortunately the body–brain connection is often ignored in everyday health care, where presenting symptoms are quickly addressed with antibiotics, anti-inflammatories or anti-anxiety medications. Such 'quick fix' solutions ignore the complex relationship between physiology, emotion and behaviour. An alternative approach is offered by Stephen Porges (2001) and colleagues, whose research into the *polyvagal system* is informative in highlighting how the autonomic nervous system operates through a hierarchy of three response systems. Each system has evolved at a different stage of evolution and each system is associated with a specific behavioural strategy. It is desirable that, in everyday settings, we operate within the most-evolved 'social engagement system' where we react to stress through communication behaviours (e.g. facial expression, vocalisation, listening, self-soothing). However, early childhood experiences may have produced traumatic experiences where the use of such a system has not been responded to, in which case more primitive systems may be dominant – both during times of stress and in everyday settings (which may, of course, be perceived as stressful). These more primitive systems instigate 'fight or flight' mobilisation behaviours (stage two) or, if the stress is still not relieved, 'freeze' immobilisation behaviours (stage three). Each of these response systems utilises different parts of the brain and body and the prolonged use of systems two and three can have detrimental effects on our physiology, as well as on our social relationships (see also Cozolino, 2013).

In my work with families, I am often aware of repeated digestive and bowel-related problems, stomach pain, headaches, migraines and a propensity to pick up infections due to a depleted autoimmune system. Being overweight or underweight, with all the attendant health implications, is also common, since using restricting food or compulsive eating plays a role in self-soothing and self-medicating against the daily experiences of trauma. Such observations make sense in the context of polyvagal theory and the findings of the ACE study.

Self-medicating behaviours

When feeling stressed and anxious, young people rarely seek medical attention. Indeed, young people often avoid attempts to explore their emotional health and well-being for fear of stigma and beliefs that it will not help (Rickwood *et al.*, 2005). It is also likely that they don't realise that they are overly stressed or traumatised because the sensations produced by trauma are familiar to them: it is how their system is set most of the time until they get insight into ways to 'turn it off'. A young child may pull their hair out and find it absorbing and soothing; they might pick at their skin, or find that lighting fires brings them a momentary sense of relaxation and 'wellness' which they want to repeat. Young people are also adept at discovering ways to alleviate their anxiety and stress – some healthy, others risky. Illicit drug-taking and drug addiction is strongly associated with experiencing adverse childhood experiences (Dube *et al.*, 2003) and, as commonly reported by practitioners working with adolescent-to-parent abuse, substance misuse is a frequent co-occurring issue (see Howard and Holt, this volume). Parents also alleviate their stress and anxiety in unhealthy ways but this is more difficult to ascertain as parents are less likely to tell me, presumably for fear of being judged – fears which may be compounded if there are anxieties about safeguarding and what such behaviours might be assumed to indicate in terms of their ability to parent and meet their child's needs.

Education and work

Most children and young people I have worked with have struggled in mainstream education because it is too much for their already-exhausted, overstretched survival system. As Music explains:

> If one has been subjected to constant trauma it is possible to become chronically hyperaroused, sensing danger everywhere and rarely calming down. Hyper-aroused and multiply traumatised children can seem like soldiers still trying to fight a war that in fact ended long ago.
>
> (Music, 2011: 93)

They are in such a state of 'hypervigilance' of any perceived threat from any direction that they are constantly on the edge of *fight, flight or freeze*. This makes it difficult to be able to settle and concentrate long enough to learn or remember anything within a mainstream school setting. Many of the children and young people I worked with had been excluded from school on a 'revolving door' basis, often culminating in a permanent exclusion and having to start over in another school.

Parents would regularly be asked to attend meetings in schools and experience the shame of being seen as the struggling or failing parent and their child as being a 'problem' (see also McDonald and Thomas, 2003). Daily reports of difficulties and unacceptable behaviour increase tension and frustrations at home (see Holt, 2009). Children's needs were often addressed at an intellectual level by adults who cared but who had limited understanding of trauma and attachment needs. It is not standard practice to access training and information about trauma in education in England, yet educational professionals were tasked with 'raising standards' as a priority for every child. Of the school-leavers I have worked with at Wish, they all finished at school with very few qualifications, yet were clearly intelligent young people.

Housing and a sense of 'home'

Having somewhere safe and secure to live is a basic human need. I have worked with families experiencing temporary homelessness and living in a refuge, hostel or a bed and breakfast, which is so stressful it leaves little room for anything else (see Paquette and Bassuk, 2009). A largely predictable living environment soothes us and allows us 'down time'; experiencing one's home and neighbourhood as 'unsafe' is extremely stressful, especially if this is also one's experience in (pre)school. Growing up and staying in a house where there has been violence and abuse is also likely to trigger latent trauma and anxiety. When families have weathered the storms of repetitive daily trauma (such as domestic abuse), their shared experience of a tense, unpredictable and threatening environment is often bound by unspoken 'secrets' and a level of parental denial or ignorance about what the children saw, heard and sensed. Post-domestic abuse, living with the same people who saw and heard terrible things can of itself be traumatic because our brains and bodily systems mirror the emotional states of those we are closest to. When everyone is responding within a more primitive response system (i.e. fight, flight or freeze), things can get confrontational and dramatic over the smallest issue.

Poverty and finances

For the majority of families I worked with, money was an ongoing daily concern. Most families comprised single-parent households and many relied on state benefits and/or low-paid work, combined with caring responsibilities for other family members. While work for many parents gave them something to focus on other than an abusive family life, often work brought a great deal of additional stress as parents could not always be present when children arrived home from school and college: parents would often tell me that they felt guilty and exhausted from doing low-paid, demanding jobs and then having to cope with family life. Lack of money produced other anxieties, such as concerns that their children had to be in work or at college, as non-engagement had financial implications for the household budget. This would often be a cause of conflict, especially when young people were asking for (or taking) money for cannabis, cigarettes or alcohol: conflict often happened when parents tried to say 'no' (see Eckstein, 2004).

For families who operate at a high level of stress and anxiety, budgeting is rarely a priority and is not something they find easy to do, which can lead to additional pressures. This is something I have seen in most traumatised families I have worked with over the years, and have personal experience of: the less money you have, the more stressful life is, as there is a daily sense of 'impending doom' because if the cooker, fridge or washing machine breaks down it will be catastrophic because there is no money to replace it. Financial decisions become (more) 'emotionally driven' and this rarely leads to sensible decisions. However, time and again I have also observed an impressive resourcefulness within these families despite unexpected and multiple demands, including the supporting of others outside the immediate family who are experiencing even worse financial difficulties.

Distractions and additional pressures

Young people

For many of the young people I have worked with there have been other 'distractions' which have felt like additional pressures but which can also bring comfort to their lives. Intimate relationships, friendships and peer groups offer young people periods of stability and contentment, but stress and anxiety are produced when there are 'fall outs' or when there is peer pressure to take risks in a variety of forms. Problems for their siblings at school or in the neighbourhood also impact some of the young people, who are generally highly protective of their family if they come under 'attack' from others. Most young people I support have 'absent' parents in their lives. In some cases there was contact with the absent parent, predominantly fathers, and this brings a whole raft of issues: some of the fathers are alternatively needy and rejecting; some are substance-dependent and rarely maintain regular contact with their child, and have little intention of building a relationship with them or meeting their emotional needs. There is also the general distraction of being a young person experiencing physical, emotional, cognitive, social and sexual changes as the body and brain approach adulthood. Adolescence can be a period of immense adjustment and this can bring additional complexities and stress into a young person's life. This can make young people seem 'distracted' and prone to 'over-reaction', even when they are not experiencing the effects of trauma. However, at this period in the young person's life, the brain is more malleable and 'open', so that – with the right kind of support – change can be transformational.

Parents

It has always been of interest to me how parents, who are raising several children alone, all with complex needs and difficulties, are also often involved in caring for others in their extended family or circle of friends. I have sometimes suggested to them that it could serve as a 'distraction' because, if they always had somewhere to be or someone to help, they could avoid their own trauma and emotional needs. Another common theme involves parents' attempts to manage complex child contact arrangements for some or all of their children. This usually brings them into some kind of regular communication with abusive ex-partners (and/or their ex-partner's families) which, in turn, can trigger past trauma, thereby increasing stress levels while being emotionally distracting and draining for them.

Furthermore, the parents I work with often have complex relationships with their own parents. Sometimes this means they are still caught up in trying to please them and gain their 'approval', which often plays out in them taking on additional caring responsibilities by attending to their health needs. Others have an 'oscillating relationship' with their own parents, which, while it sometimes seems fine, can quickly become 'confrontational' and may involve sporadic periods of 'fall out'. Some parents were being constantly undermined by their own parents, especially with regard to their parenting of the young person presenting difficult behaviours. However, in some cases there are no parents alive or available to offer either support or criticism. This can leave parents isolated and without any respite from their own childcare responsibilities.

A trauma-based approach to working with adolescent-to-parent abuse: my practice

Most of the families I have worked with in my professional life have had some experience of early childhood trauma, mostly (but not exclusively) via domestic abuse and violence in the home. Therefore, I have become increasingly curious about the brain and how it is impacted by trauma as an explanation for inter-generational violence. My inability to accept that children or young people just do 'bad things' or are simply 'naughty' has led me to seek a more scientific explanation which I can feed back to the parents I work with. This enables them to consider their child's behaviour from a different perspective – one where they do not have to feel that they have failed them. From the research literature on brain development, trauma and attachment, I offer families insights into what they have to contend with and overcome, and why their journey has been so hard. I also believe that parents should be given every opportunity to enjoy bringing up their children, and so I spend a great deal of time exploring ways to enable parents to emotionally connect with their children so they get more of the pleasure and less of the stress. I applied this approach to my work at Wish for a Brighter Future.

Attachment between child and caregiver impacted by trauma

Early attachment underpins every aspect of our daily life and I integrate an awareness of this into all areas of my intervention work. Indeed, problems with attachment formed a major part of my hypothesis about what lay at the root of adolescent-to-parent abuse. Bowlby's seminal work on attachment and loss (see Bowlby, 1940, 1969) produced a fascination with how we are shaped by our earliest relationships and the notion that our first attachment bond forms a 'blueprint' for all subsequent relationships. Attachment was defined by Bowlby as the 'lasting psychological connectedness between human beings' (1969: 194) and it is what drives us all as our survival and well-being depend on it. The primary attachment bond is formed in the first year of life through closeness between the infant and her/his primary caregiver. This closeness requires both physical proximity *and* emotional proximity and, as Shemmings and Shemmings explain: 'the fact that a parent is nearby physically does not assuage attachment needs unless he or she is emotionally present' (Shemmings and Shemmings, 2011: 20).

A parent may be emotionally absent for many reasons. For example, if a parent is living in an abusive relationship where she has to focus intently on the needs of her abuser in order to 'survive', and is having to second-guess what might 'upset' him and provide an excuse for emotional or physical assault, there is little time and emotional resource left to emotionally engage with an infant. Loving and playful interaction with a child might be a dangerous 'luxury' which could ultimately threaten a mother's survival, as this might be interpreted by an abuser as neglectful of her partner's needs. All of the families I worked with at Wish had experienced a range of complex trauma, much of it relating to domestic abuse. This is often part of a 'toxic trio', operating alongside mental illness and substance dependence. The presenting difficulties, of a young person being physically and/or emotionally abusive towards their parent, often relates to their earliest childhood relationships with their parent(s) or carer(s) and, in turn, those of their parents with their earliest caregiver(s). I make this bold statement as it is all I have ever discovered, in the course of 20 years of working with families, when I have explored their history back through the generations. Research in the fields of childhood attachment and trauma show that having a parent who, for a wide range of reasons (such as substance dependency, post-natal depression, high anxiety, depression, or other mental illness), finds it difficult to emotionally engage with their infant tends to leave their baby overwhelmed with feelings that it cannot regulate.[4] This causes the infant to experience high levels of stress and an infant's brain has no capacity to soothe itself: it needs a mature, emotionally attuned brain to do it for it so as to enable the infant's system to learn how to do it for itself. Leaving babies to 'cry it out' may eventually mean they get 'knocked out' by high levels of stress hormones, but it is not because the baby has calmed down. As Bruce Perry explains:

> Without predictable, responsive, nurturing and sensory-enriched caregiving, the infant's potential for normal bonding and attachments will be unrealized. The brain systems responsible for healthy emotional relationships will not develop in an optimal way without the right kinds of experiences at the *right times* in life.
>
> (Perry, 2001: 3)

For the infant's earliest attachment needs to be met, the infant may have had to do something extreme to produce adult interaction. This may mean screaming so that a stressed or angry adult may come and attend to them, and if no one attends to them, they may simply withdraw from the world. Without the experience of soothing, the developing baby's system is bathed in stress hormones, meaning that they are more likely to be tense and alert and find it harder to cope with life's little ups and downs. There is a wealth of published research linking the role of trauma with the disruption of early attachment relationships between mother and child (e.g. Lannert *et al.*, 2014) and with eliciting traumatic stress symptoms in infants (e.g. Scheeringa and Zeanah, 2001). Indeed, as van der Kolk *et al.* explain, 'it is often difficult to distinguish the problems that result from disorganised attachment from those that result from trauma: They are often intertwined' (van der Kolk, 2014: 118).

What has this got to do with adolescent-to-parent abuse? If a young person does not know how to be in a relationship with a parent, if they are not secure in the fact that they can get their needs met as a matter of course, particularly their emotional needs, then they will be more anxious and erratic. Without an internalised, underlying rhythm to the child–parent relationship and an unspoken focus on emotional connection, they are more likely to experience the relationship as stressful, and it may produce a sense of anxiety. As a young person develops through childhood and adolescence, they will try – often with their most primitive response system – to make sense of their life and those cognitive, emotional, social, sexual and physical transitions, but this will be particularly difficult if they cannot get support that is soothing, kind and consistently accepting of their struggles. Such support is unlikely if their own transitions are met largely by parental stress and emotional overload. Furthermore, if their response system flicks into *fight* as its preferred strategy when it feels under threat, especially if this also happens to their parent, then there is every chance that conflicts and confrontations could get physical as both protagonists operate in a more primitive *fight* response mode. If a young person has spent a lifetime watching this play out between the adults around them, it is perhaps even more likely to happen, especially as most parents I have worked with tell me that, once they verbally 'lose it', they find it hard to stop.

My direct work with young people and their parents

Traumatised parents need support to care for traumatised children and young people. Providing such support requires good self-awareness, an understanding of what is going on for the young person, empathy, the ability to prioritise the relationship with the young person, to be able to teach them how to self-regulate their emotional state and to offer calmness, emotional connection and, at some stage, correction and exploration of a different way forward. Explosive outbursts and behaviours can sometimes 'just happen' when a young person is very stressed and traumatised, as they are more easily triggered, but often there are signs leading up to it which can be learned by them and by their parent. Likewise, for an exhausted parent bearing the brunt of daily life and abuse it is very difficult for them to step back, take care of themselves and learn to monitor their own emotional and physical well-being, yet this is vital.

The great thing about working with Wish is that innovation is welcomed so long as it is led by the needs of the families. Young people can receive support without the engagement of their parents, although this is not my preferred approach as the issues are clearly posited within the child–parent attachment relationship. Thus, in those families where there is the least parental engagement, one finds the least amount of change (and, in cases where the families increasingly disengaged from working with me,[5] some aspects of the young person's life (such as behaviour in school) deteriorated).

Once I began working with families referred to Wish, my hypothesis of the abuse having its roots in attachment, childhood trauma and brain function was quickly affirmed. On inviting young people and parents to share their journey to this point, I heard many stories of having lived around repeated exposure to domestic violence as children, young people and into adult relationships. However, the impact of this repetitive trauma on child–parent relationships, parenting capacity, mental and physical well-being, access to learning, relationships with peers and siblings and the aggression and verbal abuse being visited by the young people on their parents had not been heard and needed exploring.

Sessions with the young people

My work with young people (and often their siblings) was underpinned by two key elements: (i) a genuine curiosity about them and their journey to this point, and (ii) an understanding of how our brain is shaped by exposure to stress and fear when it is developing, to enable them to better understand themselves, their behaviour and their relationships. I tried to meet once a week with the young people, although this was not always possible: I was working part-time and the young people had other commitments and were sometimes difficult to contact. However, weekly sessions were recommended for at least the initial sessions as it was a time of building trust and showing the young people that I could be trusted and was committed to working with them. I provided individual sessions with young people outside of the family home, at whatever location they felt able to go to – sometimes in school if that was easiest for them. Our time was often spent exploring and unravelling events in their daily lives; it often concerned practical issues, such as identifying college courses, developing CVs, discussing employment options and finding ways they could access other forms of support. This led them into relating current issues to earlier events in their lives and past influences. We would piece this all together in an attempt to make sense of the here and now in terms of their behaviour towards others and its emotional impact, and what they wanted in life. I always included an explanation of *MacLean's triune brain* (MacLean, 1990; see Music, 2011: 86–87) in a way that was accessible and memorable[6] and most of them said that this made a real difference. They found it useful to understand how their *reactive survival brain* could 'hijack' their thinking, as they then felt more able to see that this was something they could develop an awareness of and take care of.

All the young people were interested in working and living a different life from the one they currently had, and I often found that non-directive work such as writing CVs together and discussing the young person's qualities, abilities and ambitions was useful in helping them to identify a positive future. By exploring the *fight, flight and freeze response* and looking at their *reactive survival brain*, I would share techniques and information about how to manage stress levels in daily life and how to recognise signs in the body that would indicate that they were getting tense. I would also offer insight into what it might feel like for their parents too. We would examine past incidents where they lashed out either physically or verbally and explore how they had been feeling, both emotionally and physically (e.g. very stressed, tired, worried about something else, craving nicotine or cannabis); if they had stored resentment about an earlier incident with their parent; what had been the outcome for their parent, their siblings and themselves; how it had felt and what they wanted to happen instead. I found all the young people very committed to the process, but for those whose parents would not engage, they struggled to take things on and carry them alone.

Sessions with the parents

My work with their parents was also underpinned by two key elements: (i) a genuine curiosity about how they had reached this point of crisis in their relationship with their child, and (ii) an understanding about how the brain is shaped by early childhood experiences of trauma, in the hope that this would offer them an explanation of the young person's behaviours and of their own reactions to them so that this could form the foundation for a new way of being able to relate to each other. My focus was clearly on their child–parent relationship but also on a deeper understanding of what trauma does to the brain and body and how to live more comfortably with this to reduce confrontation and harm.

With the parents, working with them was often a more complex process because they might have practical needs and additional challenges relating to their other children, current or ex partners, finances and unresolved or misunderstood trauma from adult relationships and/or their childhoods. Changes in the young people's behaviour and attitudes were often easier to see than changes in their parents. This is perhaps unsurprising because, as mentioned earlier, it is easier to embrace change when we are younger as the brain is more malleable. Parents often could not acknowledge changes in the young people as they often seemed anxious about another issue relating to them: many of the parents had ingrained beliefs, fear systems and many pressures in their daily lives which were often consequences of their own trauma and which they bravely battled on a daily basis while bring up their children.

I also tried to offer weekly sessions to the parents and with them I would try to explore what childhood had been like for them and how these experiences may have impacted on their adult life and relationships, and on their relationship with their child(ren). I offered explanations for their child's behaviour in the context of childhood trauma and explored the use of kindness and compassion rather than enforcing boundaries, offering rewards and using 'consequences'. What lay behind such an approach was the need to prioritise a more caring, empathetic relationship with their child which was based on mutual respect. Parenting that relies upon extrinsic tools, based on the understanding that 'you get this if you please me, you lose that if you don't', can lead to more confrontation as this puts the parent in the position of having to be *more powerful* than their child and having to *enforce* consequences. This is not something I would recommend as it can inflame an already precarious situation and, in the long run, it teaches the young person little except that they need to learn to comply or be *more powerful* (which too often replicates what they will have already observed in abusive adult relationships which were neither close nor healthy).

A primary focus of my work is to address self-regulation: the more primitive the response system is when reacting to fear or threat (which can be a result of early childhood trauma), the more it will trigger strong reactions and emotional de-regulation which can quickly produce illogical confrontations. I offer a simple explanation of the three systems of the brain and explain how early experiences, if they are traumatic, might lead to the more primitive systems dominating. This is likely to mean that the 'fight or flight' mode is triggered by the merest hint of anything threatening and this can interfere with all aspects of child and adolescent development, relating to others and daily life. As the parents also often present with similarly reactive survival brains, I also explore with them the importance of their own calmness and how to regain it, which response system they need to operate within to react calmly and how they could then make better decisions and emotionally connect with their child. Parents learn breathing exercises and phrases to repeat to themselves when feeling stressed. We also look at how parents might reduce their commitments, simplify their daily life, learn to self-care, be aware of the power of offering emotional connection in bite-sized pieces to their child, correcting behaviour once everyone is calm, and how to work with their child to 'problem-solve' situations. None of this is easy to do but it is essential for a different outcome. For some parents, understanding their own and their child's trauma enables them to see things differently: they are less likely to see the young person's behaviour as being about trying to have power over them or hurt them and more about their child's reaction to previous trauma which needs them to respond calmly by offering emotional connection and co-learning.

The results have been variable and are ongoing. In most families there has been a clear reduction or end to the violence and abuse. Some young people are now in college or employment and report that they feel they 'get on better now' with their parents. For some young people, cannabis use has reduced and they appear more optimistic about their futures. For those where the relationship with their parent has not changed greatly, there are further issues and difficulties. It is a big 'ask' for young people and their parents to change what they do and how they view each other's behaviour after so many years of living together, but when they are able to do this, things improve. The more the parents are able to see their child differently and the less reactive they can be themselves, the better the outcomes.

Summary

There are no magic wands in this work. Simply teaching a young person or parent how to control their behaviour and consider each other's feelings is a start. Developing a clear understanding of how their early experiences have brought them to this point and how that can be addressed as a priority in their daily lives is a vital addition to this work. Young children are driven to connect with their main carers in order to survive, and this desire for closeness is very present in all of the young people I have worked with. We are all emotionally driven relational beings and we do better when we are closely connected and have a sense of 'mattering' to those we care about. Indeed, Elliot's (2011) research identified the importance of 'mattering' as a key risk factor in adolescent-perpetrated family violence. Every child feels more regulated, less stressed and can get on with being a child or young person if they have an internalised sense of 'mattering' and being good enough to the people who matter most in their lives. If they have grown up with this, then life and relating to others will have been easier to contend with. Thinking back to the concept of 'attachment', a child's earliest experiences of being 'good enough' to be emotionally soothed and responded to are pivotal to helping them manage stress and anxiety and developing warm and rewarding relationships.

It is very early days when it comes to fully understanding and supporting families who are devastated by daily experiences of adolescent-to-parent abuse. It is encouraging that there is now a global 'curiosity' about this issue, because the more 'parent abuse' is talked and written about, the more parents may feel they can reach out for the support they need and deserve. As I learn more about this issue, alarm bells ring when young people are referred to as 'perpetrators' and adolescent-to-parent abuse is positioned under the 'umbrella' of domestic abuse and viewed as 'learned behaviour'. Having worked with families impacted by a range of trauma and abuse for many years, it seems to me that such labels do not enable either the child or the parent to imagine or create different ways of 'being' in a relationship together, which, unlike an intimate adult relationship, is a lifelong relationship. The lens of trauma and complex attachment must be the lens through which we view and support this disconnect, which makes itself known in the troubling and painful experience of adolescent-to-parent abuse.

Notes

1 National Society for the Prevention of Cruelty to Children (NSPCC)
2 I had to end work with one family after two weeks because it emerged that there was continuing domestic violence in the household between adults. This meant that continuing with my own intervention work would create risks of further victimisation for the parent and the young person.
3 Soon after establishing their new remit in 2011, Wish were approached by an adoption support service, as well as adoptive parents looking for support. After a full exploration of the needs of adoptive families, the difficult decision was made to only work with families where abuse is towards birth parents. Our research suggested that offering such support would bring an additional layer of complexity and would require a specifically tailored response which could not be undertaken at that time due to funding and capacity limitations. However, there is a real need for support in these contexts as physical and emotional abuse are frequently part of daily life for adoptive, kinship and foster carers (see Selwyn *et al.*, 2014).
4 This can be illustrated by watching the *Tronick Still Face Experiment* on YouTube, which shows a baby whose brain is wired to expect its mother to interact and be playful. When the mother's engagement abruptly stops and the baby is presented with his mother's 'still face', we see the baby trying everything to recreate what feels familiar and comfortable. When this does not work, the baby becomes deregulated both emotionally and physically and he becomes upset. However, very quickly once the parent starts to interact again the baby appears happy and relaxed as that is what its brain 'knows' and is soothed by. It can be useful to show this clip to parents when working with them to elicit discussion about the role of attachment and emotional responsiveness.
5 Family disengagement from the intervention process tended to happen when they conceptualised the problem as 'within' the young person who needed 'fixing'.
6 See www.parentingposttrauma.co.uk/blog/introducing-the-meerkat-brain-a-simple-understanding-of-a-scared-brain

References

Anda, R. F., Felitti, V. J., Bremner, J. D., Walker, J. D., Whitfield, C. H., Perry, B. D., Dube, S. R. and Giles, W. H. (2006). The enduring effects of abuse and related adverse experiences in childhood. *European Archives of Psychiatry and Clinical Neuroscience, 256*(3), 174–186.

Anda, R. F., Butchart, A., Felitti, V. J. and Brown, D. W. (2010). Building a framework for global surveillance of the public health implications of adverse childhood experiences. *American Journal of Preventive Medicine, 39*(1), 93–98.

Bowlby, J. (1940). The influence of early environment in the development of neurosis and neurotic character. *The International Journal of Psychoanalysis, 21*, 154–178.

Bowlby, J. (1969). *Attachment and Loss. Volume 1: Attachment.* London: Hogarth Press.

Centers for Disease Control and Prevention. (2014). *The ACE Study* [online]. Available from: www.cdc.gov/violenceprevention/acestudy/ (Accessed 17 January 2015).

Cozolino, L. (2013). *The Social Neuroscience of Education: Optimizing Attachment and Learning in the Classroom.* New York: W.W. Norton & Company.

Dube, S. R., Felitti, V. J., Dong, M., Chapman, D. P., Giles, W. H. and Anda, R. F. (2003). Childhood abuse, neglect, and household dysfunction and the risk of illicit drug use: The adverse childhood experiences study. *Pediatrics, 111*(3), 564–572.

Eckstein, N. J. (2004). Emergent issues in families experiencing adolescent-to-parent abuse. *Western Journal of Communication, 68*(4), 365–388.

Elliott, G. C., Cunningham, S. M., Colangelo, M. and Gelles, R. J. (2011). Perceived mattering to the family and physical violence within the family by adolescents. *Journal of Family Issues, 32*(8), 1007–1029.

Holt, A. (2009). (En)gendering responsibilities: Experiences of parenting a 'young offender'. *Howard Journal of Criminal Justice, 48*(4), 344–356.

Lannert, B. K., Garcia, A. M., Smagur, K. E., Yalch, M. M., Levendosky, A. A., Bogat, G. A. and Lonstein, J. S. (2014). Relational trauma in the context of intimate partner violence. *Child Abuse & Neglect, 38*(12), 1966–1975.

MacLean, P. D. (1990). *The Triune Brain in Evolution: Role in Paleocerebral Functions.* New York: Springer.

McDonald, T. and Thomas, G. (2003). Parents' reflections on their children being excluded. *Emotional and Behavioural Difficulties, 8*(2), 108–119.

Music, G. (2010). *Nurturing Natures: Attachment and Children's Emotional, Sociocultural and Brain Development.* London: Psychology Press.

Paquette, K. and Bassuk, E. L. (2009). Parenting and homelessness: Overview and introduction to the special section. *American Journal of Orthopsychiatry, 79*(3), 292–298.

Perry, B. D. (2001). Bonding and attachment in maltreated children: Consequences of emotional neglect in childhood. *Child Trauma Academy Parent and Caregiver Education Series, 1*(4). Retrieved from: www.childtrauma.org/images/stories/Articles/attcar4_03_v2_r.pdf (Accessed 28 December 2014).

Porges, S. W. (2001). The polyvagal theory: Phylogenetic substrates of a social nervous system. *International Journal of Psychophysiology, 42*(2), 123–146.

Rickwood, D., Deane, F. P., Wilson, C. J. and Ciarrochi, J. (2005). Young people's help-seeking for mental health problems. *Advances in Mental Health, 4*(3), 218–251.

Routt, G. and Anderson, L. (2015). *Adolescent Violence in the Home: Restorative Approaches to Building Healthy, Respectful Family Relationships.* London: Routledge.

Scheeringa, M. S. and Zeanah, C. H. (2001). A relational perspective on PTSD in early childhood. *Journal of Traumatic Stress, 14*(4), 799–815.

Selwyn, J., Wijedasa, D. N. and Meakings, S. J. (2014). *Beyond the Adoption Order: Challenges, Interventions and Disruptions.* London: Department for Education.

Shemmings, D. and Shemmings, Y. (2011). *Understanding Disorganized Attachment: Theory and Practice for Working with Children and Adults.* London: Jessica Kingsley.

van der Kolk, B. A. (2014). *The Body Keeps the Score: Brain, Mind, and Body in the Healing of Trauma.* New York: Viking Press.

5

RESPONDING TO FILIO-PARENTAL VIOLENCE

Family dynamics and therapeutic intervention[1]

Roberto Pereira

Introduction

Filio-parental violence (FPV) is understood as repeated, aggressive patterns of behaviour directed towards parents or other adults *in loco parentis*. It involves conduct that is physical (e.g. striking, pushing, throwing objects), verbal (e.g. repeated insults or threats), and/or non-verbal (e.g. threatening gestures, breaking valued possessions) (see Pereira, 2006: 7–8). As in other Western countries, professionals working in this field suggest it has become significantly more common in Spain over the past decade. Judicial records support this claim, which show a 400 per cent increase in the number of accusations made by parents against their children during the period 2007–2012.[2] Furthermore, a recent prevalence study in the Basque Country, which collected data from 2,700 adolescents over a 4-year period, found that 14.2 per cent of adolescents admitted acts of severe psychological violence against their parents during the past year, while 3.2 per cent had committed severe physical violence (Calvete *et al.*, 2013).[3] These data were corroborated by the young people's parents, although the parental data indicated a slightly lower percentage of aggressive attacks.

This apparent sudden increase in FPV in Spain made an immediate impact on the public institutions that deal with adolescents and their families, which includes the Ministry of Health, the Ministry of Justice, and Social Services. For example, the Department of Juvenile Justice found that when tribunals applied domestic violence laws to cases of FPV, the courts used restraining orders on young people who had been accused by their parents. This involved forcing them to leave their homes and ordering them to stay in custodial institutions or those run by Social Services. However, the detention centres in operation up to that point were designed for juvenile delinquency outside the family home, and the profile of those involved was very different from those young people who were accused of FPV. The urgent need to find alternative solutions gave rise to the development of the *Euskarri Centre for Intervention in Filio-Parental Violence*.[4] Euskarri is an outpatient health clinic based in Bilbao, northern Spain, and was established in 2005 as part of a training school in systemic family therapy.[5] Initially, cases were referred to Euskarri by youth court judges through an agreement with the Department of Juvenile Justice in the Basque Government. However, cases are now referred by a range of other agencies, including Social Services and Health Services, as well as through private referrals (which are now the most common form of referral). The Euskarri team is made up of qualified psychotherapists (principally psychologists) who are specifically trained to work with FPV, and who lend their services to the Centre on a part-time basis. On average, 24 treatment requests are received each year, of which approximately 60 per cent progress beyond the assessment stage. It is standard practice to use co-therapy, and, with the family's consent, all sessions are recorded on video. We currently have a collection of 90 complete video-recorded treatments. This chapter is informed by our work and research at the Euskarri Centre.

'New' FPV

FPV is not a new phenomenon: it remained hidden for a long time as it tended to be conceptualized as just one of the many conflicts that might be presented by a family with other, seemingly more serious dysfunctions. One decisive factor explains its sudden appearance on the public stage: the emergence of a 'new' violence profile among apparently *normal families* – that is, violence on the part of children who present no other problems. In such cases, there is no previous involvement with psychiatric or social services, families are not considered to be socially excluded, and the child's violence may extend over a period of time within the family context but will show little or no violence outside of this environment. Indeed, in other contexts they may even exhibit highly well-adjusted modes of conduct. Consumption of intoxicants is common, but no more so than is typical of adolescents of that age (see Romero *et al.*, 2006). This group is the primary cause of the large increase in cases coming to the attention of the justice system.

The traditional form of FPV presents as an additional issue linked to a more significant one, such as a severe psychopathological disorder or mental deficiency. Alternatively, traditional FPV may be a response to child neglect or experiencing or witnessing domestic violence. In contrast, 'new FPV' (henceforth NFPV) involves acts of filial aggression which constitute the core of the problem. In such cases, NFPV is the presenting complaint which brings about the consultation and/or 'coercive' referral. This very rarely occurs in traditional FPV, where the reason for referral is frequently something other than violence.

All forms of intra-familial violence involve the quest for power and control in the family: both child abuse and intimate partner violence are attempts to gain power and control over the family members being mistreated. There are no immediate, specific goals being sought for which the violence is employed – these come at a later stage as a result of using the power won by the violence. However, in one respect NFPV is crucially different from these other forms of family violence because certain specific objectives are being sought and violence is used as a means of achieving them. The feeling of power and control comes afterwards as a consequence of having employed this violence, which is reinforced through its continued use. Thus, there are always specific objectives in play in cases of NFPV: the acquisition of physical objects, greater privileges or greater freedom of action (see Pereira, 2012).

Theoretical background

Our intervention work is informed by the systemic-relational model, which understands problems, conflicts and symptoms as the consequence of interactions between individuals *qua* members of human systems.[6] The psychopathology appears as an expression of dysfunction in the relevant system, generally the family. It is therefore in this familial interaction that the causes of these problems should be sought and where solutions may be found. This is not to suggest that there is no responsibility involved in using violence: there is, and it always belongs to the person who resorts to violence. However, if we do not understand the dynamics of the familial relationships, we will find it difficult to understand the apparently contradictory patterns of conduct that occur in such cases. Violent conduct often seems to be something inexplicable, yet such behaviour does make sense within the context of each family's relationships, and it is this (apparently illogical) rationale that we must try to understand to be able to intervene successfully. Moreover, it is particularly this form of intra-familial violence where we can most clearly see that the roles of 'victim' and 'aggressor' are interchangeable, and the person who is labelled as the tormentor at one point may quickly become the victim (see Perrone and Nannini, 1997).

This approach does not fit within a legal framework. From the standpoint of the judiciary, which analyses one or several acts which are presumably *criminal*, it is normal to designate one aggressor and one victim. The machinery of justice may then pass its judgment and sentence. In this way, the legal perspective involves a linear construction of events, which privileges a relationship of cause and effect from a uni-directional perspective. However, if we apply this same approach to the study of human behaviour, which is always interactive and always influenced by the behaviour of those around us, we find that much human conduct is impossible to explain. How can we understand why the person labelled as the victim would actively contest the restraining order that had been issued for his or her own protection? How can we understand a victim's repeated minimization of violent conduct? How can we understand violence which targets the parent who is looking after the aggressive child, instead of the parent who pays the child no attention or was absent during his or her upbringing? In order to understand these types of behaviour, we must introduce the idea of *circularity*: reciprocal and continuous interaction among participants in a sequence of communication (or of conduct: communication and conduct are identical; see Watzlawick *et al.*, 1981).

Here, cause and effect overlap, as each behavioural action is the effect of the previous one, and the cause of the following one.[7]

Family dynamics in cases of New FVP

Dysfunctional family dynamics are typical of NFPV, in terms of both the family's structure and their relationship processes. The structure of these families presents clear dysfunction in three principal areas (see Harbin and Madden, 1979): the hierarchical organization and establishment of rules; the protection of the family image, and separation and fusion. Each of these will now be discussed in turn.

1. Hierarchical organization and establishment of rules

The lack of a clear hierarchy is the principal characteristic of how these families function. The absence of a hierarchy is constant, whether the family is multi-violent or not, and whether it is a single-parent family or a family with other parents present. The difficulty of establishing rules and limits is the most common characteristic identified during consultations, along with a family's admission of failure in this area and a request that somebody from outside the family take on the task of reinstating the hierarchy. In these families, we find that one of the parents – and at times both parents – has abdicated from his or her parental role and has therefore stopped acting as a parent. Alternatively, it may be that rivalry between two parents prevents them from establishing rules, or perhaps the rules they create are ineffective. This presents no obstacle to them almost unanimously attributing their abdication of their child-rearing role to the personality and violent conduct of the child. 'There's nothing we can do' is the leitmotiv that not only conceals the parents' inability to take on a role in the hierarchy, but also often gives rise to a lack of collaboration when it comes to tackling the problem: the line of thought being that *if others solve the problem, then it wasn't really impossible, which means that I was partly responsible for it*. The failure or refusal to set up a hierarchy that enables rules to be established and enforced is linked to several factors which we have found to be common in families that experience NFVP: *triangulations*, where the child's support is sought by one of the parents to form an alliance (common in cases where the spousal relationship is marked by conflict); a *fused relationship* between the violent child and one of the parents (characterized by an excessive closeness or intimacy); and *conflicts and rivalry between the parents*, as neither of them allows the other to establish rules consistently.

2. Protection of the image of the family

In cases of NFPV, the image of the family – including both the image of the parents and that of the violent child(ren) – is in a poor state. The parents' feeling of having failed in bringing up their child, their shame at being assaulted by their child and their desire to protect the family image results in almost all families denying the seriousness of the aggression and minimizing its effects, even when its impact is public and unmistakeably clear. This constitutes a serious impediment for the proper prevention and treatment of NFPV, since families only come to the consultant's attention when the acts of aggression become public for one reason or another – perhaps because they require medical attention or because instances of this aggression occur in other environments, such as at school or among friends. Such a deterioration in family circumstances brings a reaction which attempts to project an image that is entirely in opposition to the truth; as a result, much weight is given to the family myth of peace and harmony. This is a fairly common myth in all families, but it is maintained in these particular families despite all available evidence, until the violence transcends the walls of the home.[8] To hide what is happening, a family secret is built up: certain topics are avoided and family members stop talking about situations and modes of behaviour that might bring the family myth into question.

Keeping this secret brings with it a fear of confrontation or open discussion regarding violent conduct, the minimization of this violent conduct and its effects, and a refusal to take consistent action to counter it: *if nothing happened* then it makes no sense to take any unusual measures, or to ask for help, or to report what happened, or to consult any specialist resource. As it becomes increasingly difficult to keep these events secret, contact with the outside world becomes less and less frequent: communication with the extended family and with friends is restricted, excursions outside the house become less common and any conversation that might touch upon 'intimate' matters is avoided. This behaviour results in a growing sense of isolation, which is often actively encouraged by the violent child who sees it as evidence of the growth in his or her power. All of this helps promote a further increase in violent conduct. Isolation, then, is a helpful condition for keeping the secret, but this creates a vicious circle which makes the problem worse. However, it is understandable: few things offer a more complete destruction of our shared family ideal than the inversion of the natural order implied by a child striking a parent.

3. Separation and fusion

In his description of young aggressors, Cyrulnik (2005: 75) noted that, of all the adolescents he has encountered who mistreat others, none have had the opportunity to experience the effect of separation. In almost every family treated at Euskarri, there is evidence of *emotional fusion* occurring between the aggressor and the parental victim at a previous stage in the lead-up to the onset of violent behaviour. 'Emotional fusion' refers to a very close relationship which does not allow the individuals involved to have different emotions and interests. Such a relationship is very satisfying in terms of mutual support and reassurance, but it does not allow for differentiation and makes autonomy very difficult to achieve. It is an intense relationship and highly emotionally charged. If maintained for a long period of time, emotional fusion tends to create problems.

The existence of such a relationship may be surprising, especially if the violent behaviour is firmly established and the parent–child relationship is badly damaged by the time the case is examined. However, emotional fusion appears in the vast majority of cases, even if it is necessary to look many years into the past. This kind of relationship is easier to observe in single-parent families, since the child often takes the place of the parent's spouse, resulting at times in a pseudo-incestuous relationship: confidences are exchanged, which may be very intimate; the two individuals involved seek mutual support, go out together, and share a bedroom or a bed (see Mouren, Halfon and Dugas, 1985).

For a while, this kind of very close relationship will suit the individuals involved – the parent finds support, company and comfort during a difficult period, while the child obtains a privileged relationship with the parent, helps the parent to feel better and gains advantages over any other siblings there may be.

However, once the child reaches adolescence, such a close, fused bond may feel oppressive, limiting or dangerous to the child, and in this context the emergence of violence may be understood as a primitive attempt to manufacture distance and find a way out of the relationship. Other benefits of violent conduct – such as power and control – are secondary concerns, and are contributory factors to the maintenance of violence, rather than its onset. The excessive proximity between parent and child also highlights the impossibility of creating a hierarchical relationship. *If my child is my friend, my support and my confidante, then I cannot put myself in a position of authority*: this often leads to the child becoming independent too soon.

The same phenomenon can occur in families where both parents are present, where the imposition of authority is blocked by parental conflict, or by abdication

---

Case study: Inés

When Inés came for consultation, we were met with a mother who had separated from her spouse, and was young and attractive. She lived with her parents and her only son, who was 18 years old, with whom she had shared a room for years and who had been violent towards her since he reached adolescence. No contact was maintained with the father and although Inés had had a 'friend' for a while, she had no plans to leave the familial home. After reporting her son's attacks, he was sentenced to stay for a period of time in a juvenile facility, but Inés arranged for the judge to allow her son to return home ahead of schedule, and he returned once again to his mother's bedroom. It took several sessions, and several attempts to remove the son from that bedroom (all of which were blocked by Inés), for us to find out that the house had three bedrooms, but two of them were occupied by grandparents, who had slept separately for years.

from the parental role. This lack of authority, or its inconsistent use stemming from the parents' inability to develop and uphold clear rules, allows the child significant room for manoeuvre. However, this requires that the child take responsibility for his or her conduct sooner than is normal, and while at first such children may seem delighted to have greater control over their own activities, they soon realize what this means in terms of responsibility – particularly in cases of *parentification*, where elder children find themselves forced to take care of their younger siblings. Such a realization can be frightening, but it is difficult to turn back the clock because parents may be unwilling to take back that responsibility, or they may be prevented from doing so by their ongoing spousal conflicts. Furthermore, such children have no great freedom when it comes to deciding how much distance there should be between them and the parents they depend on for their survival. While they need some distance, especially during adolescence, they lack the means or ability to regulate that distance in a peaceful way – without resorting to conflict – if their parents do not help them in this. However, emotional fusion is not only found where there is spousal conflict. In many cases, an emotional distance between the spouses can lead to the emotional fusion of one spouse with the soon-to-be violent child. Again, this may lead to the seemingly paradoxical, yet common, situation where violence is targeted towards the parent to whom the child is closest, as the child begins to seek more space and assert their individual identity. In such cases, the parent who has chosen the child is reproachful of this: the child's desire to develop his or her own life is seen as an attack on their relationship and the parent fears being left alone after 'choosing' the child over their spouse. Violence thus appears as a 'primitive attempt at separation' (see Mouren, Halfon, and Dugas, 1985: 294). In this sense, the child is pushing out against the allied parent, saying 'give me space, go away, don't love me so much'. But in light of the parent's reaction, and the widening of the scope of the child's power, the violent behaviour is repeated. It is the perception of the 'benefits' that violence brings which perpetuates and sustains it.

The onset and continuation of violent conduct

The process by which violent behaviour begins may be outlined in Box 5.1.

While the fused relationship is initially desirable to both individuals involved, its emotional intensity makes it very difficult to mature and problems begin to surface when the individuals involved do not develop at the same time, and one individual rejects the distance that the other attempts to put between them. The continuation of violent behaviour is based on the benefits that such behaviour brings. As stated above, any form of aggressive conduct within the family is an attempt to seek increased power and influence and this occurs in all forms of intra-familial violence. However, in the case of NFPV, the quest for power is not only related to control, but also to the achievement of certain objectives: being able to come home at the desired time, having more money to spend on things, being able to decide when and what to eat – in short, complete freedom of action.

Box 5.1 The onset and maintenance of violent conduct towards parents

Conflict/distancing between parents

↓

The child becomes part of the conflict

↓

Triangulation

↓

The allied parent sides with the triangulated child

↓

Fused relationship with the allied parent

↓

Difficulties encountered when pursuing separation and autonomy

↓

Conflict between emotional fusion and the desire for autonomy

↓

Violence appears as a desperate solution allowing the child to distance him-herself

↓

Appreciation of the benefits produced by violence leads to its perpetuation

The child not only attempts to gain power over the parents, but will also try to reduce potential competition and restrict the parents' movements and communications. The goal is to avoid any external interference that may endanger the power which the child has built up, as well as trying to frighten the parents into defenceless submission.

As time passes, the parent–child relationship becomes less strong and of lower quality, and relationships with siblings deteriorate likewise. Parents learn to ignore their child's negative behaviour in order to avoid confrontation and so the child is forced into more and more extreme behaviour in order to strengthen his or her power (see Omer, 2004).

The goals of the aggressive child are the same as those of political and social violence: exerting control through fear by repeatedly employing violent actions with an increasing level of threat, which, according to the framework for political and social violence proposed by Carlos Sluzki (2002), ends up producing a kind of *blunted submission* in its victims.

Case study: Enrique

Enrique, an only child, completely absorbed all the attention of his mother, who was separated from her partner. When he reached adolescence, he began to control his mother's relationship with the outside world. He controlled her telephone calls, demanding that she cut short any calls which he considered unnecessary. He demanded that she stay in the house when it was not essential for her to leave and he answered whenever anyone came to the house, refusing any visits that he did not think appropriate.

Case study: Antonia

Antonia told us that she had decided to put a bolt on her bedroom door because of how afraid she was to sleep at night, thinking that her son would come home in an aggressive mood. 'Every time anything to do with ill-treatment came on the TV he would say to me, "You'll end up like that". I already saw ghosts at night, thinking that I was going to go mad. It was like I was standing guard . . . I was in a really bad way, and panicked . . . I've not been able to speak because of fear, lots of times.'

Communication channels steadily close – channels established with the outside world and channels within the family itself. The family isolates itself from society, not only because of the child's active sabotage of it, but because of the parents' shame and fear of the prospect of what is happening in their house becoming public knowledge, with the corresponding damage to the image of the family, as detailed above.

Therapeutic intervention

If we accept the systemic-relational model and the important role that family dynamics play at both the onset and continuation of NFPV, then the development of a relationship-orientated strategy of intervention is inevitable. This strategy should focus on the modification of this internal family dynamic: if treatment were to seek only the eradication of violent conduct – clearly an objective of primary importance – without changing how relationships in the family operate, then the most likely outcome is that the aggressive behaviour will continue, and later worsen (see Pereira, 2012). Thus, the therapeutic task involves the need to simultaneously address the three areas of family dysfunction: hierarchical organization and the establishment of rules; protection of the family image; and separation and fusion. However, intervention also needs to reconstruct the bond between parents and children, which has been seriously damaged by the violent behaviour and which often produces a blinkered perspective on events in each family member.

Interventions should not focus on the violence *per se*, since that is 'homeostatic' and such a focus will not change the rules that govern how the family functions.[9] It is necessary to *understand* the violent behaviour in as much detail as possible and to try to put a stop to it as quickly as possible. To this end, at Euskarri we use a *pact of non-violence* which is signed by all family members once the initial phase of the NFPV intervention is completed, and which sets the conditions that must be adhered to if the rest of the treatment is to proceed. As is the case with any form of intra-familial violence, intervention is a complex matter. The inherent difficulty of the problem is normally exacerbated by the urgency of the request, by the referral of the patient being compulsory (often supported by a judicial order) and by the frequent lack of cooperation from one or more parties involved. It is not uncommon to experience additional external pressures as different authorities become involved, such as Social Services, Child Health or the judiciary. It is therefore useful to have a clearly defined intervention protocol which sets out certain objectives and certain stages which are to be completed in a prescribed order. This provides a linear scale against which progress can be mapped and facilitates an evaluation of what these strategies have achieved.

The psychotherapeutic intervention we describe here is performed on an outpatient basis, and is aimed at families with children of any age, who may live at home or live in institutional or foster care settings and who repeatedly exhibit NFPV behaviours. The intervention will always begin with the family, as it is essential to obtain their cooperation if treatment is to be successful. Every session with the family lasts for approximately 75 minutes and there are two sessions per week. Treatment length time varies between 9 and 15 months, except in those cases which are referred to us from the justice system, where treatment usually lasts for the length of time stipulated in the legal judgment.

After the first family interventions, other individuals may be introduced, or the focus may shift onto different family sub-systems: the parental couple, the children, or other combinations of family members. The proposed protocol suggests an overall paradigm for intervention, which should be adapted to fit each individual case:

Starting point

- Define the goal of therapy as the wellbeing of all in the absence of violence
- Clarify that family violence of any kind is unacceptable
- Specify that the therapists' role is not to judge but to help
- Obtain the cooperation of all family members, and involve them in problem-solving.

Initial phase

The overall aim of the initial phase of intervention is to explore the specific set of questions which a case presents and offer a relational interpretation of them. The family's involvement and collaboration in this is essential, and so the therapists work with the whole family for at least the first four sessions. The initial phase closes with an 'Intervention Proposal' which is formalized by means of a 'Therapeutic Contract'. The specific aims of this stage are to:

- Provide the family with an appropriate introduction to this new context, explaining its characteristics and helping them acclimatize to it.
- Involve all family members in the discussion of problems and issues, and to obtain information from each of them.
- Make adjustments in order to accommodate and engage the family, creating an atmosphere of confidence where everyone is listened to. This will aid communication and the articulation of problems and difficulties.
- Explore the relevant problem and the familial interactions that organize around it, in order to get a clear picture of their behavioural patterns – especially those which relate to the problem under discussion.
- Verify the role of other people in the intervention.
- Explore any solutions that have been previously attempted.
- Create a 'therapeutic system'.

Regarding the violent behaviour in particular, the aims are:

- Explore the violent behaviour, without losing sight of family relationships.
- Identify repetitive interactional patterns that precede violent behaviour, exploring the role played by each family member.
- Challenge both the minimization of violent behaviour and its impact:

  - If violent conduct is *minimized*, discuss it at length – exploring its characteristics, asking why it is not seen as important, and ensuring that it is perceived as important.
  - If the role of violent conduct *per se* is *exaggerated*, look for problems that preceded it, or which cannot be blamed on such behaviour

- Clarify that violent behaviour can be controlled, but that doing so is everyone's responsibility.
- Recognize the suffering experienced by every family member.
- Be clear, direct and transparent regarding the task that the family faces, and that it will involve hearing things that are uncomfortable.
- Formalize a *pact of non-violence*, to be maintained at least for the duration of the intervention.

An essential task during this initial phase will involve identifying the psychotherapeutic context as independent from any organizations that have been involved in the case referral. While the referral may have been compulsory, it should be made clear to the family that, as far as possible, decisions relating to the course of the therapy will be taken inside the therapy room. The nature of the practitioner's relationship to the institutions which made the referral should be clearly explained. This task of defining the therapeutic context as independent is accompanied by the task of creating a *therapeutic alliance* with all family members, although special attention must be given to the designated patient, particularly in a compulsory referral.

The work done during interviews must of course be adapted to the characteristics of each familial system; however, the following paradigm is suggested to provide an orientation:

First interview

During the first interview, special emphasis will be placed on making the family comfortable, with particular attention given to the establishment of family *circularity* (see earlier). Without directly challenging the designation of 'patient' and 'symptom', attention will be drawn to any kind of behaviour or interaction which may allow this circularity to be set up. The therapists will seek a detailed account of the violent behaviour, including information on its precursors, consequences, onset, duration, others' reactions to it, the attitude of other family members, what attempts have been made to solve the problem, and so on. In doing so, it is important to draw attention to the suffering caused to all family members.

Second and third interviews

The initial aims of making the family comfortable, promoting circularity and obtaining a description of the violence will continue, if that description is incomplete. Other objectives include:

- Explore the possibility of a *pact of non-violence*, which should include everyone involved and should last for at least the duration of therapy
- Explore how the family functions in areas relating to the problem
- Construct a *genogram* in an attempt to find connections between family history and current problems, with special attention paid to any previous history of violence.

Fourth interview

Emphasis is placed on the formulation of a specific set of objectives, based on a clear account of what is being requested by the family members. In addition, the *pact of non-violence* should be formulated, if this has not been done already (see Appendix). A refusal to 'sign' this pact will prevent treatment continuing to the next phase: until the pact is endorsed, the intervention is brought to a halt at the end of this initial phase. The objective of the *pact of non-violence* is twofold. First, the act of discussing, accepting and signing the pact has a positive impact on the violent behaviour. Second, it allows the focus of any confrontation regarding violence (if the pact is not adhered to) to shift away from the interaction between family members and onto the interaction between family and therapists.

Middle phase

The aim of this phase is to establish changes in family functioning which render violent behaviour unnecessary. The plan for therapeutic intervention is developed through the following tasks:

• Develop and strengthen the therapeutic relationship
• Propose alternatives to the behaviour being treated
• Continue gathering information on how the family operates.

After the initial family interviews, the possibility of individual work with one family member may be considered, whether that is the designated patient or any other member of the family. Individual interviews will always be coordinated, and will on occasion be carried out at the same time as family interviews (which remain the cornerstone of the treatment). Individual work with a patient may have the following aims:

• Identify which external situations foster aggressive behaviours, paying special attention to the relational aspect
• Identify which internal experiences (emotions and cognitions) favour the onset or development of aggressive behaviours. This helps the individual to recognize anger and to anticipate potentially aggressive situations
• Explore areas of suffering which underpin the aggression
• Strengthen impulse control, using medication if necessary
• Work with the social network of the designated patient or that of the family, with the aim of strengthening external support.

Final phase

The objective of the final phase is to conclude the therapy and to agree on appropriate ways forward and on subsequent monitoring. Once the decision has been taken to terminate the therapy, with the agreement of the family, the therapy is assessed and the solutions which have been developed will be reinforced as a whole. Other courses of action (such as therapeutic or educational strategies) may be suggested, either for the family as a whole, or for one family member to carry out after therapy has been completed. If necessary, a report will be sent to the relevant authorities.

Specific interventions

Depending on what phase a family is at in the therapeutic process, interventions may take a particular focus – on hierarchy and rules, on the fused relationship between aggressor and victim, or on spousal conflict and triangulation.

Intervention regarding hierarchy and rules

Sometimes the family dynamic has so deteriorated that it is very difficult to work on the affected relationships. In such cases, perhaps all that can be done is to promote an acceptable form of cohabitation, intervening specifically in restoring the family hierarchy and establishing basic rules of cohabitation and respect. This focus aims to:

- Re-empower parents so that they can establish and maintain basic standards of living
- Insist that the parents must take responsibility for that task
- Work on negotiation skills
- Insist that the parents collaborate on this task and do not sabotage one another.

Intervention in the fused phase

As already discussed, in almost every case treated at our centre we have found that at some point there has been a very close relationship between the aggressive child and the parental victim, which we term *emotional fusion*. Although this kind of relationship may appear in any familial configuration, it is most commonly found where a family currently includes only one parent. If the exploration of a family's life reveals that they are currently going through such a stage, intervention will focus on:

- Investigating the emotionally fused relationship between the parent and the violent child
- Exploring boundaries
- Exploring the context/situation of the lone parent
- Examining the relationships with the parent who is not co-habitant and, if appropriate, facilitating communication with that parent
- Exploring and challenging feelings of guilt
- Finding out about any previous history of violence
- Developing interventions which are particularly directed towards facilitating separation between the fused child and parent.

Intervention in families where both parents are present

NFPV in families where both parents are present suggests the possibility of hidden or open conflict between the parents – with both sides devaluing the other – and a lack of boundaries, and/or with little effort made to establish and maintain authority. It is common to find *pseudo-mutual behaviour* (see Wynne *et al.*, 1971), where the attempt to maintain a relationship comes at the cost of approving any kind of behaviour, by any family member. Even if this behaviour is clearly inappropriate, instead of acknowledging it, pretence is maintained that there is no such behaviour: it becomes a secret or part of the family myth.

At some stage during the development of spousal conflict, *triangulation* emerges. The child's participation in the spousal conflict, along with confrontation with the non-allied parent, produces a deterioration that ultimately leads the child to ask the allied parent to choose between them ('him or me'). At such a stage, intervention should focus on:

- Exploring the parents' relationship – suggest at least one interview as a couple
- Investigating how parents will agree on how to act with their children, especially when they display violent behaviour
- Exploring boundaries and the parents' ability to impose rules
- If violence is only directed towards one parent, exploring what the other parent does when this happens
- Exploring possible secrets and family myths that facilitate the onset of violence
- If it is hidden, bringing conflict into the open and intervening in cases of *triangulation*.

Evaluating the intervention

A telephone follow-up was conducted six months after the intervention was completed. This has allowed us to gather some data regarding its effectiveness (out of 43 cases): 71 per cent of families mentioned positive changes coming out of the therapy; violence had ceased in 90 per cent of cases; the changes identified primarily involved changes in family functioning; perhaps surprisingly, there are no significant differences between families who come to therapy voluntarily and those whose attendance is compulsory (see Montes, 2013).[10]

Conclusion

The family dynamics which are evident in cases of NFPV have their origin in parental conflict, whether present or past. This conflict has certain characteristics: it lasts for a long time with no resolution and those surrounding the couple are progressively caught up in it. The distancing and antipathy produced between the parents creates an important deficit in the child's upbringing, which particularly affects any construction of a family hierarchy, and the establishment and maintenance of rules. One of the children is eventually brought into the parents' conflict (triangulation) and develops a close alliance with one of the parents. A very close, emotionally fused relationship then emerges between the child and the allied parent – this frequently occurs during a phase where there is only one parent present.

Violence initially appears as a primitive attempt on the child's part to distance him- or herself from such a close relationship. However, the benefits of violence are quickly identified by the child, who incurs no disadvantage for having resorted to violence. The parent thus becomes part of a cycle of activity that tends towards the repeated use of violent conduct, now with the parent's consent.

Intervention must involve the whole family and must address the dysfunctional rules and behaviours that generate violence. It should aim to modify the familial structure and the way the family operates so that relationships can be maintained without the need for violent conduct. Systemic family therapy offers an effective way to approach NFPV, and its results are evident – both in the cessation of violence and in the successful introduction of changes to family functioning.

Notes

1 This chapter was translated by Richard Rabone, Merton College, University of Oxford, UK.
2 For these data, see the annual *Memorias Fiscales* published by several media outlets: *El País*, *XLSemanal*, *Qué*, *ElConfidencial.com*.
3 Severe psychological violence is defined as more than 6 discrete instances of behaviour such as threats, insults, blackmail, taking money without permission etc, all occurring within the preceding six months; Severe physical violence is defined as between 3 and 5 violent episodes in the last year.
4 See www.euskarri.es
5 Vasco-Navarra School of Family Therapy: see www.avntf-evntf.com
6 For further information on the systemic-relational model, see Minuchin (1974); Salem (1990); Linares (1997).
7 In *filial–parental violence*, there is often a struggle for attributions of blame: e.g. 'if I assaulted you it is because you provoked me', 'If I treat you wrong, it's because of your aggressive behaviour', etc. The idea of *circularity* can avoid this continuous search for culprits, since it is understood that, in human relationships, all are involved in the genesis and maintenance of a particular relational behaviour.
8 A 'family myth' is a belief that is shared by all family members, which concerns their mutual roles and the nature of their relationship, as they all join together in maintaining the *status quo* (see Ferreira, 1963).
9 'Familial homeostasis' refers to the set of rules that enable the family to function. It serves to maintain the system's *status quo*: changes that create instability in the system can cause difficulties.
10 This similarity in psychotherapeutic results from families whose attendance was voluntary or compulsory has been noted elsewhere: for example, Relvas and Sotero (2014).

References

Calvete, E. *et al.* (2013). The Adolescent Child-to-Parent Aggression Questionnaire: An examination of aggressions against parents in Spanish adolescents. *Journal of Adolescence* 36 (6), 1077–1081.
Cyrulnik, B. (2005). *El amor que nos cura*. Barcelona: Gedisa.
Ferreira, A. (1963). Family myths and homeostasis. *Archives of General Psychiatry* 9, 457–463.
Harbin, H. and D. Madden. (1979). Battered parents: A new syndrome. *American Journal of Psychiatry* 136 (10), 1288–1291.
Linares, J. L. (1997). *Identidad y narrative*. Barcelona: Paidós.

Minuchin, S. (1974). *Families and Family Therapy*. Cambridge, MA: Harvard University Press.

Montes, Y. (2013). La intervención en VFP: 6 meses después, in *Jornadas sobre Investigación en VFP*. Bilbao: Universidad de Deusto. Available online at www.euskarri.es (Retrieved 4 September 2014).

Mouren, M., O. Halfon, and M. Dugas. (1985) Une nouvelle forme d'agressivité intra-familiale: les parents battus par leur enfant. *Annales Medico Psychologiques* 143 (3), 292–296.

Omer, H. (2004). *Nonviolent Resistance: A New Approach to Violent and Self-destructive Children*. Cambridge: Cambridge University Press.

Pereira, R. (2006). Violencia filio-parental, un fenómeno emergente. *Revista Mosaico* 36, 8–9.

Pereira, R. (ed.) (2012). *Psicoterapia de la VFP*. Madrid: Morata.

Perrone, R. and N. Nannini. (1997). *Violencia y abusos sexuales en la familia. Un abordaje sistémico y comunicacional*. Barcelona: Paidós.

Relvas, A. P. and L. Sotero. (2014). *Familias obligadas, terapeutas forzosos: la alianza terapéutica en contextos coercitivos*. Mexico City: Morata.

Romero, F. *et al.* (2006). *La violència del joves a la família*. Col·leció: Justicia i societat; 28. Barcelona: Centre d'Estudis Jurídics i Formació Especializada, Generalitat de Catalunya.

Salem, G. (1990). *Abordaje terapéutico de la familia*. Barcelona: Masson.

Sluzki, C. (2002). Violencia familiar y violencia política. Implicaciones terapéuticas de un modelo familiar. In D. Friedman (ed.) *Nuevos paradigmas, cultura y subjetividad*. Buenos Aires: Paidós, pp. 351–371.

Watzlawick, P. *et al.* (1981). *Teoría de la Comunicación Humana*. Barcelona: Herder.

Wynne, L. *et al.* (1971) Pseudomutualidad en las relaciones familiares de los esquizo-frénicos. In C. Sluzki (ed.) *Interacción familiar*. Buenos Aires: Tiempo Contemporáneo, pp. 111–153.

Appendix

Contractual pact of non-violence

Family therapy is a collaborative process which requires certain conditions to be fulfilled in order to allow effective communication, expression of emotions, etc. Therefore, it is essential that the following attitudes and behaviours are displayed: listening to others; mutual respect; avoidance of any provocative action, threats or violence which may impede or prevent the free expression of feelings or opinions.

Given my interest in collaborating and participating in this process, I hereby undertake:

* to avoid any kind of violent behaviour, whether that is physical or verbal, for as long as the course of therapy lasts; and
* to avoid behaving in any way which might provoke or foster any such violent behaviours on the part of any other family member.

Any failure to adhere to the terms of this pact will be addressed within the sessions and may lead to therapy being terminated.

In Bilbao, _____ (date)

Signed: _____

_____

_____

_____

PART 2
Contexts for intervention

As explained in the Introduction, work with adolescent violence and abuse towards parents can take place in a number of kinds of contexts, and these different contexts are likely to shape working practices. One kind of context is the organisational setting. The problem of adolescent violence may come up in the caseloads of those who work in mental health, domestic violence support and in youth justice, among other settings. Each of these organisational contexts will operate within their own relevant legislation, operational procedures and practice guidelines, as well as within their own institutional norms and values, and these factors will both limit and liberate practitioners accordingly. A second kind of context is the regional and national context where practitioners find themselves. This context will shape family configurations, meanings and practices; national and regional legislature and policies; and cultural norms and values about violence, families, adolescence and harm. Finally, a third context, which intersects with the other kinds of context, concerns those aspects of personal and family life that make people who they are. Often termed 'variables', such contexts include gender, 'race' and ethnicity, age and relationship status of family members, sexuality and dis/ability, social class and myriad other relational identities. Such contexts shape both the nature and meaning of the abuse and violence experienced and the ways in which professionals work with it.

This section takes this wide definition of 'context' to explore how it may differently shape our understanding of, and our work with, families. In the first three chapters, practitioners describe their work in this field within a range of organisational settings and national/regional locales to offer insights into their professional practice as they identify successful intervention strategies and challenges encountered along the way. In Chapter 6, *Latesha Murphy-Edwards* draws on her professional experiences as a clinical psychologist working in a child and adolescent mental health service in Invercargill, New Zealand. In Chapter 7, *Ester McGeeney*, *Fiona Barakat*, *Gjori Langeland* and *Shem Williams* describe their development of

Yuva while working within a domestic violence support agency in London, UK. Yuva is a specialised intervention for adolescent violence towards parents and was developed in response to increasing demand for such a service. In Chapter 8, *Kristin Whitehill Bolton*, *Peter Lehmann* and *Catheleen Jordan* describe their development of the Youth Offender Diversion Alternative (YODA) program, a unique university–court partnership that enables the local court to offer a specialised social service for young people charged with offences against their parent(s). In the following two chapters, analysis of context takes a different focus. In Chapter 9, researchers *Kathleen Daly* and *Dannielle Wade* analyse detailed casenotes from six restorative justice conferences that featured cases of adolescent-to-parent violence. Applying a systematic analysis, the authors explore how dynamics of gender may be implicated in family contexts, types of violence, explanations for violence and disclosure practices. In Chapter 10, *Jo Howard* and *Amanda Holt* offer a review of existing research and practice to identify a range of contexts that require particular consideration when working in this field, including working with intergenerational abuse, adoption, culture, dis/ability and social class, and addressing co-occurring issues such as mental health problems and substance misuse. In the final chapter, the editor identifies areas where there is consensus across the volume and reflects on what challenges remain for developing work in this emerging and important field of family intervention.

6

RESPONDING TO PARENT ABUSE IN NEW ZEALAND

Delivering interventions within child and adolescent mental health services

Latesha Murphy-Edwards

Introduction

My first clinical experience of a young person abusing his parents came early in my career in the mid 1990s and took me by surprise. The client, John, was a 15-year-old male referred to the service with a major depressive disorder. He was from a seemingly stable and happy two-parent family and was reportedly well liked by his peers and doing well at school. John would come to sessions, always with his mother, Pam, at his own request, and would politely engage in discussion. I recall he was very softly spoken; indeed, I sometimes struggled to hear him. John spoke of several forms of stress in his life to which he attributed his low mood, including a deep sense of inadequacy. This was despite being an all-round high achiever. Although John engaged well in the therapy sessions, he was struggling to make progress, and his mood remained low. On the day of our eighth appointment, John and Pam arrived at the clinic and I immediately noticed that Pam had her right arm in a cast. Naturally I enquired about the nature of her injury. A long silence ensued while Pam and John exchanged glances. Eventually, Pam began to speak, but she only got as far as explaining that the injury had been sustained during a 'family argument' before John loudly interrupted, yelling 'Shut up. I mean it. Just shut up' before storming from the office.

I was shocked by John's behaviour, never having heard him use that tone of voice, let alone speak to his mother in that way. Immediately I felt concern that this dramatic change in behaviour might reflect a significant deterioration in his mental health. However, Pam, now in tears, explained that this was how John always behaved towards her at home, and that her injury was the result of him grabbing and twisting her arm. She further explained that this was not the first time he had physically harmed her, and that verbal and emotional abuse had been a daily experience for both her and her husband for the past 5 years. I vividly recall how Pam immediately apologised for speaking of this problem, explaining 'I didn't want to say anything, but when you asked, I just couldn't lie to you.' Of course, I tried to reassure her that talking about the abuse would help, and that I would be available to support her and John to overcome this problem. However, despite making another time to meet, neither Pam nor John returned to the clinic. Pam contacted me on the morning of our next appointment to cancel, stating that 'John was feeling much better', and they did not wish to continue with therapy.

To be honest, I felt a sense of relief, largely because I had not detected this issue of interpersonal violence in the home and I felt deeply foolish. There had been many opportunities to do so, and in hindsight, several *red flags*, which I had simply not paid enough attention to. I was particularly affected by Pam's comment about not being able to lie to me, which left me regretting that I had not asked the right questions much earlier in therapy. This experience highlighted just how ill-prepared I was at the time to ask about parent abuse, let alone offer an intervention to support this family. I wondered how many other cases of this form of family violence I had missed. Eager to avoid doing so again, I turned to the literature for information about parent abuse and specifically for models of assessment and intervention. There was very little to be found and what was available came from other parts of the world and seemed to have little applicability to the people I was seeing in my role as a clinical psychologist working in a child and youth mental health clinic in Invercargill, New Zealand.[1]

My interest in the phenomenon of children and young people abusing their parents continued to grow, largely because I was now enquiring about this issue and hearing numerous accounts of parent abuse from my clients and other practitioners. By the time I started my doctoral research,[2] which explored child- and youth-perpetrated domestic property violence towards parents, I had met many parents reporting abusive behaviours, which ranged from name-calling to assaults with fists and weapons. I was convinced that this was a serious problem and deserved the attention of researchers and practitioners, yet little focus had been given to this form of family violence. Indeed, mine was to be one of the first New Zealand investigations of parent abuse (Murphy-Edwards, 2012). The design of my study offered the opportunity to interview 14 parents affected by parent abuse and to explore their beliefs about the causes of this problem. Participants also shared the many ways they had been impacted by the abuse. I am indebted to the courageous parents and caregivers who provided their stories, as each has informed my practice.

In this chapter I share my experiences of working with young clients who behave in abusive ways towards their parents, along with several findings from my doctoral research into this problem. It is a phenomenon that I call *parent abuse* and I consistently and deliberately use this term, both in my clinical practice and in writing. This term has been criticised for creating confusion, as some will assume that parent abuse refers to parents behaving in an abusive manner towards children, and many researchers and practitioners prefer terms such as 'child-to-parent abuse' that clearly identify both the instigator (the child) and the target (the parent) of the violence.

Yet terms like *child abuse*, *partner abuse* and *elder abuse* are all regularly used in New Zealand and do not seem to create similar confusion. I suspect the discomfort some people have with the term reflects their difficulty accepting that parents can be victimised by their children. Therefore, persisting with the term *parent abuse* reflects my deliberate stance to maintain a well-accepted template for describing interpersonal violence in this country. I am also mindful that the term *parent abuse* has been criticised for being too strong and threatening. Although I would agree that the word 'abuse' can be confrontational, I have found that in many cases, adopting the term *parent abuse* can have a very powerful and beneficial impact. In short, yes it sounds serious, because it is serious.

What follows is a brief description of both the problem of parent abuse in New Zealand and of the mental health setting in which I practise, as a means of contextualising my clinical experiences of working with parent abuse. I then discuss assessment and treatment issues that arise when working with this complex and challenging problem, with a particular emphasis on identifying and managing risk.

Parent abuse in New Zealand

Family violence remains one of New Zealand's most pervasive social problems. This is despite increasing national focus on the issue through various media campaigns, anti-violence action by many statutory organisations, and improved police procedures for dealing with, and recording, family violence (Families Commission, 2011). The most significant effort in recent years to reduce family violence has been the 'It's not OK' campaign – the product of a collaboration between the Ministry of Social Development and the Families Commission, in association with organisations including the New Zealand Police and various community groups. The campaign, launched in 2007 by the Taskforce for Action on Violence within Families, aims to promote social change by encouraging people to talk about family violence and take action to prevent it. Evaluative research has been undertaken throughout the campaign to assess both impact and effectiveness, and findings suggest that the campaign is making a significant difference by both raising awareness and encouraging action (Point Research, 2010). However, while the New Zealand government recognises parent abuse in its definition of family violence,[3] family violence initiatives tend to focus on adult-perpetrated forms of violence, and parent abuse falls quite some way down the list of priorities in terms of policy guidance, funding and resources. Some progress has been made with the publication of a pamphlet titled 'Parents can be victims too' – an addition to the selection of brochures and resources developed by the 'It's not OK' campaign team.[4]

There has been no research into the prevalence of this problem in New Zealand families: agencies such as the New Zealand Police do not routinely record, collate or analyse reported incidents of parent abuse. Routine screening is now a key component of family violence initiatives in many statutory and community organisations. For example, all practitioners employed by the New Zealand government to deliver health services are expected to participate in family violence training, in order to learn ways of asking about violence in the home and to provide support to those who disclose this concern. All of New Zealand's 20 District Health Boards (DHBs) receive government funding to appoint family violence coordinators who are responsible for providing this training and for ensuring the implementation of the *Family Violence Intervention Guidelines*, published by the Ministry of Health (2002). Yet, here again, the emphasis continues to be on partner violence and child abuse. Parent abuse is seldom considered, even by those working in agencies with a focus on children and young people with behavioural and emotional problems.

Parent abuse and mental illness

Across New Zealand, clinics known as Infant, Child and Adolescent Mental Health Services (ICAMHS) offer free, outpatient interventions to young people (0–18 years) suffering with moderate to severe mental illness. Every year, one in four of New Zealand's young people are estimated to experience mental health problems, with around 7 per cent suffering from diagnosable mental health disorders that have a serious impact on their social, emotional and academic or occupational functioning (Mental Health Commission, 2011). As a result, the demand on services is high.

Most commonly reported disorders are mood and anxiety problems, disruptive behavioural disorders (such as *oppositional defiant disorder* (ODD) and *attention deficit hyperactivity disorder* (ADHD)) and substance abuse problems (our clinic primarily uses the *Diagnostic and Statistical Manual* – Fifth Edition (DSM-5) as a diagnostic classification tool). ICAMHS will also see a number of young people suffering with serious psychiatric illnesses such as *schizophrenia*, although these disorders are relatively rare. Some of the young people who attend ICAMHS will have multiple problems, including behaving in ways that are harmful to their parents and other family members. Cases of co-existing mental illness and abusive behaviour present unique challenges to the practitioner.

Many mental health conditions can lead to family interactions characterised by extreme tension and conflict. In my experience, some problems are more likely to be associated with parent abuse, particularly externalising disorders such as *oppositional defiant disorder* (ODD) and *conduct disorder* (CD).[5] However, as demonstrated in my first case study, parent abuse may exist in the families we least suspect. Young people with internalising disorders such as depressive illnesses and anxiety problems can also engage in abusive interactions – most commonly verbal or emotional abuse, but sometimes physical violence. However, the precise role that mental illness plays in shaping aggressive behaviour in young people is unclear, and debates in this field often conflate notions of 'mental illness' with 'aggression' in a way that contributes to the stigmatisation of people with mental health problems. In my clinical experience, most young people with mental disorders do not behave violently towards others and, of those who do, factors other than their mental illness are likely to play a significant role in their behaviour.

Several research studies have explored the influence of mental health problems on parent abuse (e.g. De Lange and Olivier, 2004; Ghanizadeh and Jafari, 2010).

In my own research, a number of parents reported that their abusive children had required interventions for problems that included depression, anxiety and substance abuse and, in such cases, the presence of emotional symptoms can influence the type and frequency of their abusive behaviour. However, the relationship between parent abuse and mental health is a bidirectional one in that the abusive behaviour can also influence the young person's emotional wellbeing, which presents an additional challenge to mental health practitioners. To complicate matters further, in some cases parent abuse takes the form of a young person intentionally adopting behaviours that suggest mental illness but are in fact designed to worry, upset or undermine their parents. Examples include withdrawing from the family, choosing not to speak, and refusing to perform daily activities such as getting out of bed, washing or eating. The ICAMHS clinician needs to consider the context within which these behaviours occur and the presence or absence of other symptoms we would expect to see in a child suffering from a serious mental health concern. Behaviours that occur only in response to, say, parental limit-setting would suggest the child has more control than he or she would like the parent to believe.

Defining parent abuse during therapy

When I am concerned about parent abuse occurring in a family, I give the problem a name (*parent abuse*) and then I introduce a definition of this problem, focusing on the **intentional** nature of behaviour that has the **purpose** of assuming power and control over a parent. It is important to distinguish between behaviour towards parents that is deliberately employed to cause harm, from actions that are impulsive, inconsiderate or irresponsible but not intended to be harmful. Furthermore, when thinking about parent abuse I do not generally include aggression directed at parents that is associated with serious psychotic disorders such as schizophrenia, developmental conditions like severe autism, or other situations where young people have diminished control over their behaviour.

I have found it helpful to encourage the client, whether it is the young person, the parent, or both, to formulate their own definition of the issue as it exists within their home. I like to capture parents' beliefs about children's behaviour, particularly what they consider to be normal versus abnormal, or acceptable versus unacceptable, behaviour. Specifically, I enquire about standards around the use of bad language, yelling, threatening, hitting and breaking objects. This sort of conversation can assist parents to reflect on their experiences and begin to identify what behaviours are concerning to them and harmful.

Family members are often surprised to learn of the term parent abuse and its definition. Parents may report: 'I have never thought of her behaviour as being abusive, I guess I have just put it down to being normal teenage behaviour and put up with it.' Collaboratively formulating a definition of *parent abuse*, and indeed simply giving the family a language to speak of the problem, can have a very powerful effect. Several participants in my doctoral research described how hearing the term parent abuse for the first time prompted a realisation that what they had been experiencing was not what other parents would consider normal or acceptable behaviour, and it was time to respond differently.

Making sense of parent abuse: techniques for opening a dialogue

Once it has been established that a young person's actions are harmful and abusive, it is useful to explore everyone's perceptions of why the behaviours occur. For some parents, the abusive behaviour can be so inexplicable that a mental health explanation is the only one that makes sense: as one mother commented: 'There must be something wrong with his head. Why else would he behave in this way?'

A question I am regularly asked is: 'Does the depression [or other disorder] make him act in this way?' This is not an easy question to answer because, in some cases, the mental health condition may be associated with an emotional dysregulation which contributes to externalising behaviours such as aggression. However, in the majority of cases, while associated with the symptoms of the mental health condition, *parent abuse* cannot wholly be explained or excused by the illness. Indeed it would be both misleading and unhelpful to think of the disorder as causing the abusive behaviour. This type of thinking can diminish the child's personal responsibility for the violence and their motivation to make necessary changes. Furthermore, it may lead to parents tolerating a range of behaviours that they might not otherwise have accepted in their home.

Reports by young people of 'just losing it', and parental descriptions such as 'he's not able to control himself' and 'it's like watching *Jekyll and Hyde*' are frequent. I have also heard numerous descriptions of abusive episodes that cannot be recalled by the young person after the act. One mother explained: 'When she calms down I ask her to tell me why she did that, and she just can't remember. It's like she blacks out.'

These unusual 'symptoms' are highly concerning for parents, who may see them as confirmation of a serious mental health problem. The clinician hearing these reports needs to consider each carefully, and investigate the presence of other symptoms that might indicate a serious neurological or psychiatric disorder. When amnesic or dissociative-type experiences[6] occur in isolation from other symptoms, and present only during or after episodes of parent abuse, it would be reasonable to conclude that these complaints may be the young person's attempt to avoid responsibility for his or her actions.

When trying to make sense of their children's mental health problems and misconduct, parents may struggle to accept the idea that the behaviour is purposeful. But it is an important point to make if progress is to be made with respect to improving the child's behaviour in the home. Beyond this, parents can be supported to recognise that their young person's recovery from mental illness will benefit from changes to the present family situation, particularity the cessation of all forms of parent abuse. I work with parents to build their understanding that a safe, cohesive, non-violent home, led by strong, warm and consistent parents or caregivers, will optimise their child's chances of recovery. Conversely, making allowances or tolerating abusive behaviour will not benefit the young person in the long term.

When parents or their children have difficulty letting go of the idea that parent abuse is 'caused' by a mental health disorder, I find it helpful to engage in a functional assessment process as a means of demystifying episodes of abuse. I invite young people to answer questions like:

- The last time you threatened to harm your mum, what was going on for you?
- What did you want your actions to achieve?
- Looking back, could you have decided to take a different approach?

These types of questions are designed to assist the young person to reflect on the intentions of their actions and on their decision-making ability before and during an episode of abusive behaviour. In my experience, enquiries like these can promote insight in young people but do need to be delivered in the context of a trusting therapeutic relationship to avoid defensive responses.

Another approach is to encourage the young person to reflect on their interactions with people outside of the family, particularly during situations that have been upsetting or frustrating:

- How did you respond when your teacher prevented you from going outside to play basketball?
- Your reactions to your teacher saying 'no' are very different from your reactions to your mum. Why do you think this is?

Such questions can draw attention to examples that disprove the theory that the young person's behaviour is caused by a mental illness and therefore outside of his or her control. This is a useful strategy not only for discrediting this idea but also for focusing on the young person's capacity to respond in a pro-social manner.

Of course, before we begin to implement any techniques designed to assist the child and his or her family, we need to form a detailed picture of our young client and the factors that have brought him or her to the clinic. In the following section I discuss assessment issues and considerations when working with young people and their parents for whom parent abuse is a feature of family life.

Uncovering parent abuse

In some cases, parent abuse is a concern but it is difficult to expose – often because parents feel ashamed or afraid that they, or their child, will be judged harshly by others. Unfortunately, it would seem that their fears are often well founded. In my doctoral research, parents described not wishing to talk to others about their experiences of abuse because they wanted to preserve an image of their 'happy family' and/or their 'good child'. Those that did disclose the problem described receiving unhelpful responses from family members, friends and service providers who either did not see the seriousness of the issue or responded in ways that left them feeling ashamed. One mother stated: 'People perceive that if you have a child that is aggressive then you are an aggressive parent: you provide a home that is aggressive.'

Others described experiencing similar messages, conveying the premise that parent abuse only happens to parents who are blameworthy. In fact, being unfairly judged and receiving unhelpful advice were experienced by almost all of the participants, and had the detrimental result of increasing embarrassment, frustration and isolation.

However, the absence of information about parent abuse during an assessment is not always due to the family intentionally concealing the problem. Very often, family members do not raise issues because they do not see the threads that bind the various factors influencing their lives: it never ceases to amaze me what people come to the clinic expecting to discuss, and what they consider to be unimportant or irrelevant. I am certain I am not the only therapist who has experienced working with a child or family for a period of time, confident that I have a strong understanding of the situation, only to discover, sometimes by chance, that I have been missing a very significant piece of information. Often it is that missing piece of the puzzle that finally reveals the deepest and most significant of issues. In some cases, parent abuse is that missing piece.

Assessment is an ongoing process that may involve a range of data-gathering techniques, with clinical interviews providing an important source of information, particularly when the clinician has the opportunity to observe family interactions. This material then informs the development of a clinical formulation that captures the presenting problems and any influential individual, family and community factors. The challenge when working with young people who have mental health disorders and who also engage in parent abuse is finding a way to make sense of each issue while, at the same time, developing an understanding of how these problems are connected, as they invariably are. The process of carefully concept-ualising individual and family difficulties is crucial in the design of an effective intervention that is personally meaningful to all involved.

Truly comprehensive formulations are those that acknowledge the role that extrafamilial influences such as peers, media and the school environment play in the development and maintenance of mental health and behavioural problems. Culture is another important consideration, particularly when working with New Zealand youth and families. New Zealand is an ethnically diverse society comprised of Māori, the indigenous people of this country who make up around 15 per cent of the population, people of European descent, commonly referred to as 'Pākehā' (around 75 per cent), and smaller groups of people who identify as Pasifika, Asian, and a range of other ethnic and cultural groups (Statistics New Zealand, 2011). This cultural and ethnic diversity means that there is no typical New Zealand family and indeed no easy way to capture the variety of family life in this country. Rather, the construct of family can be represented in various ways, ranging from traditional

Western models of the nuclear family (whereby biological parents are largely, if not solely, responsible for child rearing), to *whanau* (the Māori-language word for family) whereby extended family groups share responsibility for raising, teaching and disciplining children. All variances along this spectrum have implications for child rearing and other aspects of family life. In my experience, most New Zealand families represent a blend of traditional Western and Māori models of child rearing.

ICAMHS clients come from differing ethnic and cultural backgrounds and so it is essential that those entrusted to work with them do so in a culturally responsive manner. For example, Drury and Munro (2008) suggest that prioritisation of 'respect for Other' and the facilitation of an atmosphere of *manaaki tangata* are essential for engagement with Māori families in mental health services. Working with parents from marginalised groups necessitates an awareness of issues such as stigma, shame or a mistrust of social agencies that may create resistance to sharing stories about family life, particularly descriptions of family violence. In my clinical practice I am fortunate to have opportunities to consult with, and work alongside, Māori mental health workers who can guide me on culturally appropriate ways of exploring parent abuse in Māori families. The importance of this was demonstrated by Ryan and Wilson (2010) whose study of Māori mothers who experience parent abuse found that those they spoke to 'felt forced to carry the secret of the violence alone' (p. 29) out of fear of further abuse and because of their experiences of *whakamā* (the Māori word for shame). I have observed that when compared to other groups, Māori parents and caregivers are particularly reluctant to disclose this problem. As one Māori mother explained to me: 'You don't want to talk about your boy being violent, because everyone just thinks, oh yeah, here we go again, another violent Māori kid, probably from a bad home.' New Zealanders frequently hear reports that Māori are significantly over-represented as both victims and perpetrators of family violence. And while this is a well-established finding (e.g. Dobbs and Eruera, 2014; Te Puni Kōkiri, 2010), I suspect that hearing this statistic time and time again has the detrimental effect of undermining the identity and wellbeing of Māori people, and causing them to be less willing to share their experiences.

Recognising risk

Risk appraisal is a central component of the comprehensive assessment and begins at the point of referral. Evaluating 'risk' (in the many forms it can take) is a fundamental area of competency for practitioners working in ICAMHS. This is because a significant proportion of the children and young people who enter our services will have experienced abuse or neglect, and many will endanger themselves through acts of deliberate self-harm, suicidal behaviour or involvement in risky activities such as drug taking. Within ICAMHS, practice guidelines for assessing and responding to risk of deliberate self-harm or suicide, along with child abuse and parental neglect, are very clear and routinely implemented.

However, assessment is more problematic in cases where the young person presents a risk to others: while there are many risk assessment tools available (each

ICAMHS has a service-specific risk checklist and recording form), most attend to a young person's history of *physical violence* and destruction of property. Risk checklists do not typically offer items designed to elicit information about non-physical forms of abuse. Consequently, risk to others is often narrowly defined as acts of physical violence, while other forms of abusive behaviour, including verbal and emotional abuse, are not routinely explored. Furthermore, risk to others is only generally considered when a client has a known history of serious misconduct and violence. This is problematic in the case of parent abuse because many of those who abuse their parents are otherwise pro-social young people with no evidence of aggression outside of the home. It is this group that may not be assessed for risk to others, because on the surface they do not appear to pose a threat of harm to anyone. Let me present two types of referrals to make this point.

Case one

Fifteen-year-old male with a diagnosis of *conduct disorder* (CD) and various reports of violence towards others. This young person's profile is going to tick a number of boxes when considering the importance of assessment for the threat of further violence, and ideally this assessment will include questions about violence towards his parents.

Case two

Fourteen-year-old female with no documented history of serious misconduct attending the clinic for treatment of *social anxiety disorder*[7] (SAD), presents a clinical profile that is less likely to prompt concern about aggression.

Hearing these two examples, the reader may be thinking *well that stands to reason: where there is violence, check the risk of more.* This is, of course, a sound suggestion, but I have used these two referral examples because they are based on two young people I have seen recently at the clinic. The young man, although often non-compliant at home and described by his mother as 'a real terror', had no history of acting in an abusive manner towards her. The young woman, on the other hand, had for several years repeatedly verbally and emotionally harmed both of her parents and had intentionally caused several thousands of dollars' worth of damage to household property. In this case, parent abuse had been a closely guarded family secret. Here again, I wish to emphasise that parent abuse can exist in the families we least expect, and could remain hidden if we do not begin to invite discussion about harmful behaviours occurring in the home.

Working with families affected by parent abuse

Aside from my own research that provides insights into parents' help-seeking experiences, there are no New Zealand-specific sources of information to inform assessment or intervention. As a result, organisational policies and practices are often under-developed with respect to the problem of parent abuse in this country. My colleagues and I often liken the task of working with families affected by parent abuse to participating in an adventure race: we need to get somewhere fast (to minimise harm), but we are often unsure of what path to take. This work regularly involves overcoming a series of obstacles, navigating unfamiliar territory, sometimes even getting lost along the way. Indeed, a guide book, complete with maps and directions, would be very useful. Unfortunately, practice manuals of this type are not available, and if they did exist, they would need to capture the vicissitudes inherent in this type of work.

I am not aware of any research that demonstrates the benefits of one treatment modality over others when intervening in cases of mental illness and parent abuse. My early clinical training was predominately focused on cognitive and behavioural therapies, although over time I have become increasingly interested in family therapies. My present method now generally combines techniques based on the principles of all three broad modalities when working with children and young people who abuse their parents, and I have had good success with this approach. However, experience has taught me that regardless of my chosen approach to intervention, my first important therapeutic tasks when addressing parent abuse include establishing *rapport*, generating *motivation* and fostering *hope*. By building strong relationships with family members, I am constructing a platform for all involved to speak openly about family matters – the good, the bad and the ugly. For some, particularly parents, the idea of sharing the bad and the ugly is simply too unpalatable or the perceived risks too great. Because various factors can influence people's preparedness even just to speak of the problem, let alone engage in a program of change, practitioners should prepare to encounter this resistance and not be put off the task of encouraging disclosure and change.

Keeping young people and their parents connected, particularly when parent abuse becomes the target of intervention, can be a real challenge. There is no one right way to proceed, but rather various options that need to be considered when designing individualised treatment plans. Therapy might involve the young person only, the young person and his/her parents, all members of the family, or parents only. A common challenge that I and colleagues encounter when working within New Zealand's mental health services for children and young people is that acceptance criteria often require a focus on the child's *problems*, and the classification of children as *disordered*. In many cases, a child's difficulties may be symptomatic of an unhealthy family system or broader social, political or cultural problems. But such concerns do not fit neatly into diagnostic boxes and so are difficult for services with restrictive boundaries, most of which are fiscally driven, to accommodate. Fortunately, once a child is accepted into ICAMHS there is scope to work with his/her parents and other family members. Very often multiple therapeutic alliances will be needed to support the young person to overcome the symptoms related to the mental health condition, and to provide assistance to other family members. In some cases, interventions will require several clinicians, working as a team, to deliver a program of change.

Do we consider parent safety?

Decision-making about the shape of therapy needs to be informed by knowledge of factors that could either enhance or diminish the family's ability to benefit from the intervention. In the case of parent abuse, risk is an important factor that needs to be carefully considered. Directly addressing parent abuse with a parent and abusive child together in some cases can expose the parent to risk of further violence when the child takes exception to what is being shared. I recall how one mother was abused by her teenage son on their way home from a therapy session. He had kicked the dashboard of her car, called her names and put his fist to her face, all before they had driven from the clinic car park. When I asked him about this behaviour, he stated, by way of an explanation, 'I was angry because she embarrassed me by talking about what's been happening at home.' Understandably this parent was reluctant to engage in further discussion about her son's abusive behaviour while he was present. She was offered appointments with another therapist to talk about her experiences of abuse and to consider ways of responding in order to keep herself and others in the home safe.

Aside from the risk of physical harm, it is also important to consider how we might enquire about parent abuse without eliciting feelings of shame or guilt in either the parent or the child. While I have a preference for working with young people and their parents together, there are times when I meet with parents on their own or, as with the case just mentioned, I may ask a colleague to do this piece of intervention, while I continue to work with the young person.

Parent and child sessions may expose parents to further emotional abuse. I have seen examples where a parent's expression of fear and shame in the presence of an abusive child results in the child being further empowered by his or her growing perception of the parent as weak and defeated. Parent-only sessions may also be necessary when the mental health of the child(ren) involved may be too deeply affected at a time when they are unable to manage this. In all cases, when ICAMHS clinicians encourage disclosure of parent abuse, they need to be well equipped to support the family with the dual aims of treating the young person's mental health concerns and preventing further parent abuse.

A strong understanding of a family's interaction style is vital when designing clinical treatment plans, and especially so in families affected by interpersonal violence because the plan will need to prioritise any risks that may arise in the implementation of the intervention. Indeed, goals for intervention need to be developed with risk as a key consideration, particularly when parents are asked to be central agents of therapeutic change. As one mother explained to me after attempting to implement a strategy I recommended with her son who had a substance problem: 'You said that I should prevent him from getting hold of more drugs, so I tried. I even stood in front of the door so he couldn't leave. He just shoved me out of the way.'

There are a variety of mental health disorders that can create stress and disharmony in the home and which heighten the risk of aggressive child-to-parent interactions. Substance abuse problems are one group. A major depressive illness can also increase family tension, particularly when the disorder contributes to the young person withdrawing or losing interest in activities such as going to school. Treatment in such cases is likely to include strategies for increasing the client's participation in daily routines. The act of waking a depressed young person and getting them out of bed in the morning can be met with much resistance. One mother I worked with some years ago spoke of dreading morning times, as her daughter would become verbally abusive when she entered her bedroom to ask her to wake up and get ready for school. Similarly, in cases of *anorexia nervosa*[8] where parental involvement is strongly recommended, volatile situations can arise, especially when a distressed young person is prepared to take whatever action is required to resist her parent's efforts to feed her. Numerous experiences of verbal and emotional abuse have been reported to me by parents of children with *anorexia nervosa*. Yet, despite causing significant harm, these behaviours are often considered by the parents and others to be inconsequential in the face of this serious illness.

In all cases, clinicians need to consider the stress their recommended interventions may place on the family. Generating honest discussion about likely responses can assist in preventing aggression by providing the young person with alternative non-abusive responses to difficult situations. For example, I might explain to my young client how an important part of overcoming his depression is keeping active, before then enquiring: 'How are you likely to react when your mum asks you to get out of bed each morning?' Equipping young people with non-aggressive strategies for coping with the symptoms of their mental health problem is an important approach in reducing episodes of parent abuse. Furthermore, it is essential to enquire of parents about their own safety concerns and support needs, and to take any suggestion of violence very seriously. Indeed, some young people will present such a serious risk to parents that they cannot remain in the home. This is a dire situation that is not easily managed, largely because there are few services available to intervene. In-patient treatment may be available in cases involving severe mental illness, or youth forensic residential care may be an option in cases of serious violence. In my research, several parents described experiencing extreme physical violence at the hands of their children, with two reporting that they feared for their lives. Hearing their stories reminded me of the importance of directly asking about any concerns that parents have for their safety and the safety of others residing in the home. Parricide is rare but does occur, and there have been several New Zealand cases of young people intentionally fatally injuring their parents or caregivers.[9]

When serious harm to anyone is imminent, police involvement will be necessary. However, I have found that parents do not always respond well to this recommendation. Several participants in my study explained that they struggled with the dichotomy of being both the *victim* and the *protector* of their children.

Clinicians need to be cognisant that parents can experience a confusing blend of love and fear that may make it very difficult to take action, such as contacting the police. When families do require the involvement of other agencies we can facilitate this by providing health and social service providers with information about the serious nature of parent abuse and the importance of responding sensitively when a parent requests assistance. This may occur in some cases, but not in all, and therefore services such as ICAMHS require practice guidelines that increase the likelihood that this type of support is offered in a consistent and coordinated manner.

Conclusion

While we cannot say with any certainty how many New Zealand families are experiencing parent abuse, it seems reasonable to speculate that a portion of children and young people who abuse their parents will access their local ICAMHS. Therefore, it is essential that practitioners are aware of parent abuse and the many serious impacts of this issue, and are prepared to invite discussion about child-to-parent interactions that are harmful. We should avoid assuming which families may be experiencing parent abuse, because as I have learned, it can occur in the families we might least expect. I have also come to realise that parent abuse is a serious and complex concern that cannot be attributed to a single cause. Rather, this problem invariably stems from the complex interaction of a host of overlapping factors, sometimes mental illness. Conceptualising multiple embedded problems, for example co-existing mental health disorders and parent abuse, requires a sound knowledge of individual and family development, context and ecology in order to design interventions that consider the needs of our young people and their parents.

Risk, in all its forms, needs to be an important consideration throughout the intervention. This is especially necessary when we are asking parents to implement treatment strategies in their homes that could increase the chances of harmful interactions between child and parent. We also need to appreciate that when we encourage parents to take actions such as contacting the police, their resistance to do so is likely due to feeling torn between defending themselves and also protecting their children. Parents, like other groups affected by family violence, require understanding and support in order to make sense of the problem and overcome self-blame, shame, and the many other impacts of parent abuse. Therefore, it is imperative that mental health services reply to all parents seeking help with this problem with policies and practices that adequately and sensitively respond to their concerns.

Notes

1   Our clinic offers assessment and treatment services to young people in the Southland region of New Zealand. Invercargill is the main urban centre, although many clients come from the surrounding rural areas.

2   I enrolled at the University of Canterbury's School of Social Work and Human Services where members of the academic staff had earlier produced the first literature review of parent abuse in New Zealand (Crichton-Hill, Evans, and Meadows, 2006).
3   As defined by the Ministry of Social Development in its policy paper *Te Rito, New Zealand Family Violence Prevention Strategy* (2002). See: www.msd.govt.nz/documents/about-msd-and-our-work/publications-resources/planning-strategy/te-rito/te-rito.pdf
4   See www.areyouok.org.nz
5   *Oppositional defiant disorder* (ODD) and *conduct disorder* (CD) are classed as 'disruptive, impulse-control, and conduct disorders' in DSM-5 and are usually diagnosed in childhood. They are characterised by problems in emotional and behavioural self-control and symptoms include irritability, defiance and/or vindictiveness (ODD) or behaviours that violate social norms (CD) (American Psychiatric Association, 2013).
6   *Dissociative experiences* refer to a sense of disconnection between consciousness, memory, identity, or perception and may include symptoms such as amnesia, depersonalisation, derealisation, identity confusion and identity alteration (Dell and O'Neil, 2011).
7   *Social anxiety disorder* (SAD) is classed as an anxiety disorder in DSM-5 and features symptoms of extreme fear of social situations which interferes with ordinary routines and everyday activities (APA, 2013).
8   *Anorexia nervosa* is classed as a 'feeding and eating disorder' in DSM-5 and is characterised by a distorted body image, excessive dieting and a pathological fear of gaining weight (APA, 2013).
9   The most recent case being that of 13-year-old Jordan Nelson, who pleaded guilty to the charge of murdering his caregiver in 2012 and was sentenced to 18 years' imprisonment (See www.stuff.co.nz/national/crime/8106900/Why-a-13-year-old-killed-his-caregiver)

References

American Psychiatric Association. (2013). *Diagnostic and statistical manual of mental disorders* (5th edn.). Arlington, VA: American Psychiatric.

Crichton-Hill, Y., Evans, N., and Meadows, L. (2006). Adolescent violence towards parents. *Te Awatea Review, 4*, 21–22.

De Lange, N. and Olivier, M. (2004). Mothers' experiences of aggression in their Tourette's syndrome children. *International Journal of the Advancement of Counselling, 26*, 65–77. doi: 10.1023/B:ADCO.0000021550. 87868.bd

Dell, P. F. and O'Neil, J. A. (eds.). (2011). *Dissociation and the dissociative disorders: DSM-V and beyond*. New York: Routledge.

Dobbs, T. and Eruera, M. (2014). *Kaupapa Māori wellbeing framework: The basis for whānau violence prevention and intervention*. Auckland, New Zealand: New Zealand Family Violence Clearinghouse, University of Auckland.

Drury, M. and Munro, T. (2008). Crisis engagement in mental health: A New Zealand Maori contribution. *International Journal of Mental Health Nursing, 17*, 317–325.

Families Commission. (2011). 2010 *Family violence statistics – good news but a long way to go*. Also available at www.familiescommission.govt.nz

Ghanizadeh, A. and Jafari, P. (2010). Risk factors of abuse of parents by their ADHD children. *European Child & Adolescent Psychiatry, 19*, 75–81. doi: 10.1007/s00787–009–0067-y

Mental Health Commission. (2011). *Child and youth mental health and addiction*. Wellington, New Zealand: Mental Health Commission: Also available at www.mhc.govt.nz

Ministry of Health. (2002). *Family violence intervention guidelines. Child and partner abuse*. Wellington, New Zealand: Ministry of Health. Also available at www.moh.govt.nz

Murphy-Edwards, L. (2012). *Not just another hole in the wall. An investigation into child and youth perpetrated domestic property violence*. Unpublished doctoral dissertation. University of

Canterbury, Christchurch, New Zealand. Also available at http://hdl.handle.net/10092/8188

Point Research. (2010). *An innovative approach to changing social attitudes around family violence in New Zealand: Key ideas, insights and lessons learnt.* The Campaign for Action on Family Violence. Also available at www.msd.govt.nz/documents/about-msd-and-our-work/publications-resources/research/campaign-action-violence-research/an-innovative-approach-to-changing-social-attitudes.pdf

Ryan, R. G. and Wilson, D. (2010). Nga tukitanga mai koka ki tona ira: Māori mothers and child to mother violence. *Nursing Praxis in New Zealand, 26,* 25–35.

Statistics New Zealand. (2011). *Demographic trends: 2010.* Wellington: Statistics New Zealand.

Te Puni Kōkiri. (2010). *Arotake Tūkino Whānau: Literature review on family violence.* Wellington: Author.

7

THE YUVA YOUNG PEOPLE'S SERVICE

A holistic approach to addressing child-to-parent violence in London

Ester McGeeney, Fiona Barakat, Gjori Langeland and Shem Williams

Introduction

The Yuva young people's service is a new initiative currently being developed by the Domestic Violence Intervention Project (DVIP) in London, UK. Established in 2010, the service works with young people using violence or abuse in their close relationships and with the partners, parents and other family members experiencing this abuse. We write this chapter as current and former employees of DVIP who have been involved in setting up and delivering the Yuva service. Drawing on personal reflections and case studies from practice, the chapter discusses the theoretical and practical principles that informed the development of the service as well as outlining the profiles of the families that we work with, the types of interventions that we have developed and the challenges we have encountered. In mapping this journey we consider questions of gender, power and responsibility in relation to child-to-parent violence (CPV) and argue that in order to address the complexity of such questions we need a holistic framework that considers the needs, rights and capacity of both parents and young people experiencing child-to-parent violence and abuse.

Developing the Yuva service: how did it all begin?

The Yuva service forms part of the wider Domestic Violence Intervention Project (DVIP). Established in 1992, DVIP is a charitable, not-for-profit organisation that was set up to deliver services to domestically abusive men and to support the women and children who are affected by this violence and abuse. Today we work with over 1,500 clients a year in London and south-east England, and we are funded from a range of sources including public sector delivery contracts and grant-making trusts. DVIP's work is based on the feminist power and control model of violence and abuse that was pioneered by the Duluth Domestic Abuse Intervention Program (DAIP) in Minnesota, USA. This model was developed in consultation with victims of abuse and proposes that intimate partner violence (IPV) is not a one-off 'explosion' of anger or frustration but is rather part of a pattern of actions used to intentionally dominate and control a partner to create an atmosphere of fear and humiliation. This early model of reparative justice was specifically formulated with three key aims: to ensure the safety of victims of domestic violence, to listen to victims and make sure that their voices and experiences are used to inform interventions and address the abuse, and to hold the abuser accountable for the abuse without bringing the victim into contact with her abuser and potentially creating opportunities for further victimisation (DVIP 2013).

DVIP's decision to develop the Yuva service in 2010 was a direct response to requests from local family support and social care services, as well as existing DVIP clients, for a specialist intervention for young people – in particular young men – who were abusing their intimate partners or family members. Practitioners working in services that were in a position to identify CPV, such as children's social care, youth offending and domestic violence support services, often reported feeling ill-equipped to address the issue because it did not fit with existing intervention frameworks (see Holt and Retford, 2013). Where these services were engaging with CPV they were largely working with either the young person using violence *or* with their parents; rarely were services able to address the needs of both parties. Furthermore, while mainstream domestic violence support services were able to support parents as victims of their child's (and often current/former partners') abuse, they were unable to meaningfully engage the young person in a programme of personal change: the dominant adult domestic violence model positions the child not as abuser but as a victim of adult violence. Such a model leaves limited scope for addressing a young person's agency in using violence towards their parents or for the complexity of a parent's responsibility for their abusive child's wellbeing.

The Yuva service was set up to address these identified gaps. Based on DVIP's core principles, it aimed to offer a service both for young people using violence in their intimate and family relationships and for the parents, partners or others affected by this violence and abuse. This model of parallel service delivery mirrored not only established best practice in adult domestic violence programmes such as DVIP, but those emerging in the burgeoning field of CPV intervention such as Break4Change, based in Brighton, UK (see Munday, 2009). The Yuva service was established using two 3-year grants from the John Lyons Charity and the City Bridge Trust. This enabled us to set up and pilot a pan-London service, to develop referral pathways and build the service model. The most readily established referral routes were with children's social care services, family intervention services and pupil referral units. This may account for the fact that the vast majority of cases (24 out of 30) referred to the services in the first year were for CPV, rather than teen relationship violence, a pattern which has continued. We also continue to have difficulties in establishing referral pathways with local youth and community services. At the end of this 3-year period, despite difficult economic conditions brought on by national and local government 'austerity' cuts to public services, we were fortunate to secure a number of small service delivery contracts from local authorities that has enabled the service to continue within particular areas of London.

Yuva clients: who do we work with?

Since its inception in 2010, the demand for the Yuva service has grown year-on-year with a 280 per cent increase in referrals over the past 4 years. We estimate that this number would be significantly higher were it not for funding being restricted to individual local authorities.[1] In the last year of service (April 2013–April 2014) we received 84 referrals for young people using violence and abuse in their close relationships, creating a challenging workload for the small team of three part-time Yuva practitioners. Eighty-six per cent of these young people were young men. Their ages ranged from 10 to 21 years, with particularly high numbers of 13–14-year-olds and 16–17-year-olds. Eighty-one per cent of these cases involved violence towards family members, 81 per cent of whom were mothers and 19 per cent of whom were fathers, siblings and grandparents. The majority (81 per cent) of the families we work with are lone-parent families and are from a range of ethnic,

Katie is a 16-year-old young woman who was referred to the Yuva service by her social worker due to concerns about her aggressive and violent outbursts at home towards her parents and younger brother. Katie lives in a damp, overcrowded flat with her parents and two brothers. Both Katie and her younger brother have been diagnosed with ADHD and her older brother has a diagnosis of ADHD, autism and learning difficulties and needs constant support. Both of Katie's parents have ongoing medical issues and receive limited support from family members with the care of their children. At the time of referral there was a Common Assessment Framework[4] (CAF) in place for Katie and her younger brother and the family were receiving family therapy. However, Katie's parents felt that the interventions made little impact as Katie continued to be both verbally and physically aggressive towards her mum and her younger brother. During initial assessment appointments, Katie's parents reported that Katie had frequent violent outbursts and had threatened to 'kill her brother with a knife' on several occasions, leading to her younger brother becoming fearful of being left alone in the house with her. Additionally, they reported that Katie had thrown objects against the wall, knocked over the wardrobe and frequently hit her mother and bullied her younger brother. When a Yuva practitioner met separately with Katie, she acknowledged that she was unhappy about her own behaviour, commenting on the difficulties she experienced in controlling herself when she was angry with her family at home.

religious and social class backgrounds. The largest ethnic group that we work with is White British, reflecting 36 per cent of referrals in the past year.[2]

The majority of referrals that we receive (84 per cent) are for young people with additional support needs, which include having a diagnosis of ADHD and ASD, experiencing problems with substances and/or alcohol, having experience of abuse (including witnessing domestic violence in the parental relationship), having caring responsibilities for their parent(s) and/or sibling(s), experiencing learning difficulties and having engaged in the criminal justice system. Furthermore, the parents often have additional support needs including physical and mental health issues, substance and alcohol problems and experience of abuse, whether currently or historically (i.e. as a child). In most cases, families have multiple support needs that affect several family members, as illustrated in the case study of Katie[3] above.

This combination of parental and child support needs can significantly compound the complexity of how best to respond to the violence: it may affect

---

Sofi and Jay were referred to the Yuva service due to Jay's violence and abuse towards his mother. Sofi had experienced 14 years of domestic violence from her husband. Her son Jay witnessed this violence and used to be very protective towards his mother, learning to be diplomatic when his father questioned him about his mother's whereabouts. When talking about the impact of the domestic violence she had experienced with her husband, Sofi described Jay as being her saviour at times of extreme violence. She says that he never even slept through the night as he was always in a state of alertness, 'ready to jump out of bed and distract his dad from attacking me'. Sofi says that Jay's father gave him a lot of power and control in the family, describing a hierarchy in which 'the father was on top, then Jay, then me'. Nearly 2 years ago, the father left the family home and went to live abroad. He now has a new wife and has made no contact with Jay since leaving the country. Sofi says that where Jay used to love his dad, he now feels completely abandoned by him. Sofi told a Yuva practitioner that Jay 'has fallen to pieces' and speaks about him with great empathy for his loss. Sofi describes outbursts in which Jay smashes and breaks everything in the house; he has punched his mother in the eye and other parts of her body, twisted her arm, kicked her and pulled her hair. Jay usually speaks to his mother in English, but when he is angry he swears at her in the language of his father's heritage, using the same derogatory and highly sexualised insults. Sofi has described him as a 'wild dog' and said that she was more scared of her 14-year-old son than she was of her violent ex-husband. She maintains that she never thought her ex-husband would kill her as he was aware of his limits and his body strength, but she believes that her son could. Sofi was arrested by the police after an incident where she grabbed Jay's arm and twisted it after he punched her in the eye.

the length of time and the number of agencies involved in providing information and support. For example, in Katie and her family's case, there was a social worker, a therapist, a respite worker, several healthcare professionals and two schools involved in the family's lives. Working in a joined-up way with such a range of agencies, each with a separate remit and theoretical understanding of the issue, represents a continual challenge for the team and for the families we work with.

By far the most common additional factor affecting the families we support is a family history of domestic violence. This is illustrated in the case study of Sofi and Jay (see above). As explored elsewhere (see Holt 2013), the correlation between a history of family domestic violence and instances of CPV does not *explain* why the violence occurs, particularly since the vast majority of young people who grow up in violent or abusive families do not go on to perpetrate violence. It does, however, have an impact on the complexity of the cases that we work with, as illustrated in the case study of Sofi and Jay.

The Yuva approach: how does it work in practice?

Initial assessment

The Yuva service primarily aims to increase the safety and wellbeing of young people and families who are living with violence and abuse. Broadly, this involves supporting families to identify and manage risk, engage in safety planning and work towards behaviour change and building positive and safe relationships. Every family that is referred to Yuva is offered an initial assessment. This involves two Yuva practitioners, each meeting separately with the young person and the parent(s) or carer. Here we use a range of techniques including the *Ecogram* and the *Abusive Behaviour Inventory* (see Table 7.2) to understand more about the lives of the young person and the parent, their relationships and support networks, and to identify the types and frequency of abusive behaviours used. Although the aim of the initial assessment is to identify a suitable package of support for the family, in practice this assessment is the beginning of intervention through supporting young people and parents to name and identify their feelings and the types of abusive or violent behaviours they are using or experiencing. Crucial to our model of practice is the close relationship and the sharing of information between the two practitioners working separately with the young person and the parent (see case study of Kay and Sam below).

Based on the initial assessment we may offer the young person and their parent/carer one-to-one tailored support sessions, possibly followed by joint work involving both practitioners and all family members. In cases in which there are multiple family members affected by the violence (such as in Katie's family), the team look at how best to support siblings and other family members alongside the parent(s). However, where resources are limited our priority is to work with the young person using violence and their primary carer. Increasingly, we are finding it challenging, and potentially unethical, to engage young people in a programme of personal change and development without the participation of their parent or carer. This is particularly the case for younger children where the absence of good communication and appropriate nurturing can make behaviour change problematic and potentially risky. Further, by engaging solely with the young person as the 'perpetrator' of violence, rather than the family as a complex site of power and control, we can become complicit in reinforcing the message that the young person is the sole cause and solution to the problem.

Key elements of Yuva service provision for families experiencing CPV

Within our service provision, there are a number of key elements which are central to our work. These are summarised in the Table 7.1 and are explored further in the following section.

Shifting agency and responsibility

A key premise of our work is the recognition that the young person has the capacity for agency and can work towards changing their behaviour. Primarily this involves choosing healthier and safer strategies for managing what they often experience as 'intolerable' feelings, such as powerlessness and despair. A young person's capacity to take responsibility for their behaviour is, however, relative to their level of cognitive and emotional development. In cases involving younger children, for example, we have found that the child will require the support of their parent(s) or other adults to help them to regulate their feelings effectively. This requires a joined-up service intervention that will support families to disentangle anger, distress and fear and balance unhealthily skewed family power dynamics through building parental agency and developing empathy between family members. Where the young person using abuse is in the older age range of adolescence (and where there are no underlying learning difficulties or mental health concerns affecting their behaviours), the onus of personal responsibility moves along the continuum, with an increased expectation of personal responsibility for one's own actions. In all cases it is important that this 'recognition' process takes place for the young person using aggressive or violent behaviour, as well as for the parent who is victimised by this behaviour.

The young people we work with may come to us with a very low perception of self-control over their physical and verbal aggression. Such comments from young people include:

'I can't control myself and all I want to do is hit her' (Sam, 16-year-old male)

'I just switch . . . I don't even realise what I'm saying . . . it's like something just takes over me and I just wanna hurt her and shut her up' (Serina, 15-year-old female)

'I have a really bad temper because of my ADHD' (Katie, 16-year-old female)

TABLE 7.1 Key elements of Yuva service provision for families experiencing CPV

Key element	Provide support for young people to:	Provide support for parents to:
Recognising agency	Recognise own agency and capacity to take responsibility. Control their aggressive, violent and abusive behaviour (in accordance with age and mental capacity).	Recognise their child's agency and evolving capacity to take responsibility and control their behaviour. Recognise their agency as parents and individuals, within a context of understanding the gendered power relations that shape their feelings and capacity to exercise this agency.
Regulating empathy and validating distress	Recognise and value their own emotions and distress. Offer empathy and validation for these emotions. Build empathy for other family members.	Empathise and understand their child's distress. Recognise and value their own distress. Regulate empathy for family members.
Exploring the function and outcomes of the abusive behaviour	Understand the function of their own behaviour (e.g. *exploring what you get out of behaving this way. How does it work for you?*)	Understand the function of their child's behaviour within the family context (e.g. *What role do they have? What are the outcomes and consequences of their behaviour?*)
Exploring more effective ways of communicating distress	Explore more effective ways of communicating distress that are safer and less destructive.	Find ways of reducing the escalation of conflict and degree of negative communication.
Contextualising the work and psycho-educational input.	Learn about relevant issues specific to your child/family (e.g the impact of DV, ADHD, mental health, triggers and responses to stress, healthy relationships, gender identity/roles, the child's education, effects of drugs, grief etc.)	

These explanations for their own violence, which place the 'cause' outside of the individual, make it difficult for the young person to exercise agency and to behave in any other way. For example, if a young man believes that he is destined to be 'just like [his] dad', he may be less likely to recognise his capacity to choose to be otherwise. Such beliefs are often reinforced by parents and other members of the family (see examples below), which can contribute to a spiral in which the young person is increasingly seen, and sees themselves, as inherently violent and without the potential to change:

'I can see that something is wrong with him, he is not normal . . . Maybe it's the smoking that is making him so aggressive' (Mum)

'He is just like his father and he knows it' (Mum)

'She is just like me, I used to have a bad temper too when I was younger' (Mum)

While such explanations of their child's behaviour may, in part, be true (smoking cannabis could be contributing to aggression, or a young person may have learnt aggressive behaviours or destructive gender norms from their father), these explanations work to reinforce the externalisation of the violent or abusive behaviour and fail to provide a framework for change.

A core aim of the Yuva service is to work with parents and young people *in parallel* to enable a shift in this attribution of responsibility. The practitioner can facilitate this process with young people by asking questions such as:

'Why did you throw the cup at the wall? Why didn't you throw it at her?'

'Why did you kick her rather than push her?'

'How long did it take you to pick up the curtain rail by the front door and walk up the stairs with it?' 'What were you thinking during that time?'

'Why did you threaten to kill her? Did you really mean it?'

'What did you want your Mum to do/stop doing?'

This style of questioning requires the young person to consider the 'intention' behind their behaviour and to identify the choices and decisions they have made about how to act and respond to difficult situations:

'I didn't throw it at her because I knew it would smash her head or something, so I threw it at wall to get her attention' (Josie, 15-year-old female)

'I kicked her because I had already pushed her to the floor, so I started kicking her' (Tyrone, 15-year-old male)

'I was thinking that I was going to hit her with the curtain rail' (Callum, 17-year-old male)

'I just wanted her to stop going on at me, I didn't really want to kill her' (Aaron, 14-year-old male)

As these responses suggest, such questions enable the young person to recognise where they exerted self-control in situations of conflict and where they chose to respond with violence. Importantly, such questions enable young people to identify and accept responsibility for their behaviours and recognise their capacity for self-control. A similar style of questioning is used with the parent: *Why do you think he threw the cup at the wall rather than at you? What do you think he was thinking at that time?* Such questions support the parent to identify their child's capacity to exercise agency and self-control in situations of conflict.

Another technique that we have found useful for enabling a shift in attribution of responsibility is to conduct a *sequence analysis* of a recent conflict situation, with the young person and/or their parent (see Table 7.2). Using this technique, the practitioner guides the client to describe, in detail, their feelings, thoughts and actions of a recent incident, asking questions such as:

> Which room were you in? Where was your Mum standing? What did he say? What did you say? Did you say that before or after you moved over to her side of the table? Who was standing in the doorway? Could your Mum leave the room? What were you feeling just before you ran up the stairs?

Used at DVIP in work with adult perpetrators and victims of domestic violence, this technique (sequence analysis) is based on the assumption that every behaviour is shaped by preceding thoughts, feelings and actions. By breaking down a moment in which a young person felt, or was perceived to be, out of control, this technique can help both the parent and the child to identify the moments in which the young person made choices and decisions about how to react to conflict and how to respond to feelings of anger, anxiety or distress.

A Yuva practitioner used the sequence analysis technique during a one-to-one session with a mother, Kay, who was engaged with the Yuva service due to her son's aggressive and 'manipulative' behaviour. Engaging in this process highlighted how her son, Sam, made her feel small and scared. When asked how anyone else might feel if they were in her shoes, Kay realised that anyone would find it scary to be on the receiving end of his aggressive behaviour. When asked to describe how her son might perceive her when they argue, she said 'he sees me as weak and not coping'. For the remainder of the session Kay and the practitioner talked about shifting this shared perception (between Kay and her son) of 'Mum is weak' to a shared perception of 'Sam's shouting is intimidating and abusive'. This was shared with the Yuva practitioner working with Sam so that he could support Sam to make a similar transition and recognise his own capacity to control and take responsibility for his behaviour. In the following session, Kay described how she found her last session very useful as it enabled her to break down a particular recent incident, identify her thoughts, feelings and reactions at that point ('I am too weak to cope') and consider how this might be perceived by her son.

Regulating empathy and validating distress

Much of the work we do with young people and their parents involves helping them to recognise and value their own, as well as others', emotions and distress. While some clients are able to identify and reflect on their emotional responses, many report feeling overwhelmed by their emotions. For example:

> 'I got so angry – everything around just went fuzzy and all I wanted to do was to smash something' (Calum, 17-year-old male)

> 'My blood starts to boil and I just explode, like something takes over me' (Halima, 16-year-old female)

> 'I get so angry, I can feel it hurting in my throat and in my heart' (Shanika, 18-year-old female)

> 'I just get a feeling of sinking and shrinking into a ball that I just want to hide away' (Mum)

One technique *Yuva* practitioners use to help young people and parents understand and regulate feelings of anger, despair, frustration and fear is to focus on the emotion and ask questions such as:

> Can you tell me more about this fuzzy/noisy/sinking sensation you had? What did it feel like physically? How long does it last? What happened and how were you feeling just before you got this feeling? When did it go away? How did you feel then? Can you recall another time when you felt like this? How was this the same or different from the previous time? What adjectives might you use to describe it?

In instances in which the young person or parent feels overwhelmed by their emotions they can find it difficult to empathise with their parent or child. Some of the questioning techniques that we might use to build empathy focus on developing a perspective, understanding and concern for others, such as:

> If your mum/child was here – how do you think they would describe how you were feeling? How did mum react? Why do you think she reacted that way? What could she have been feeling? If she was here now – how would she describe how she was feeling? Where was your younger brother at the time of the incident? How do you think he might have felt? If he was here now – what would he say he felt? Why was your baby sister crying, when you were shouting at mum?

This kind of questioning can also be done in the form of role-playing, discussion, drawings or using dolls where appropriate. It can help the client to imaginatively put themselves in the place of another, to see situations through their eyes and to identify what they might be feeling, wanting or needing. Sometimes building empathy work is extremely challenging, particularly in cases where the child or parent has a diagnosis of ADHD and/or ASD. In such cases, we use alternative approaches to support clients to develop strategies for understanding and responding to their own difficult feelings, which may involve clarifying that particular behaviours are unacceptable and teaching them how to identify these behaviours and how they could behave differently (such as walking away).

Many of the parents we work with tend to 'over-empathise' with their child who is using abusive behaviour. This may lead to a situation where the empathetic parent cannot bring herself to separate from her son/daughter in a way that facilitates psychological autonomy and ensures physical safety, due to the negative effects this might have on them. This is particularly the case where the CPV follows adult domestic violence and the mother may feel responsible for the trauma of the abuse the young person has witnessed and 'understands' their child's perception of themselves as a victim. This can be problematic when the parent's perception of her son/daughter as a victim becomes a justification for the child's behaviour, as illustrated in the case study below:

Jane is a mother of a 14-year-old daughter Shanika, who has been abusive towards her by shouting, swearing, hitting, throwing objects, and being demanding, threatening and controlling. During a session with a Yuva practitioner Jane became angry stating, 'I have had enough, I am at my wits' end, I can't take this anymore. If it wasn't for the way Shanika behaved then social services would not be involved and I wouldn't have to be here . . . how dare she treat me like this? Who does she think she is controlling my every move? She has ruined my life and has taken everything out of me . . . I want her to just go away, I never want to see her again.' At this stage, Jane was sobbing uncontrollably as if she had actually lost her daughter. She continued: 'I know what she has been through, she has suffered so much and had to grow up quickly, she was so clever in finding ways of calming her Dad down so he wouldn't hit me again. I love her so much and I couldn't live without her, she has been there for me all the time throughout my depression, the drinking and all the violence she witnessed from her Dad . . . She is so caring, she makes me cups of tea when I'm down, she advises on what to do. She is my best friend and the only person who has been with me throughout the last 15 years of my life. The truth is I need her just as much as she needs me.' The Yuva practitioner reflected back to Jane the feelings of despair, love and anger she was feeling towards her daughter and the struggle she was experiencing in managing her own and her daughter's emotions. This enabled Jane to identify a dichotomy; I love and care for my child but I hate and do not accept her abuse towards me.

In this session, Jane was able to recognise the entangled emotions and co-dependency between herself and Shanika, as well as the cognitive and emotional dissonance she was experiencing in relation to her daughter. These are common themes that we notice in the families engaged with the Yuva service, particularly those of lone-parent families. In such cases, we may use systemic questioning techniques (see Table 7.2) to disentangle and relocate which feelings belong to whom. For Jane, this helped her to recognise that 'over-empathising' with Shanika was sometimes preventing her from giving clear messages to say 'NO' and 'STOP' and 'I will not tolerate your aggressive behaviour'. Through parallel working, we were also able to explore ways of managing conflicting feelings of autonomy and dependency with both parent and child.

Exploring safer and more effective communication

Many of the families we work with communicate distress in ways that are harmful and erode their relationships with others. While aggression is very good at letting people know *I'm angry* and in getting attention, it tends to drown out other messages and concerns such as *I'm feeling hurt* or *I want you to listen to me*. For example, in the case study below, James states that he feels that shouting is the only way in which he can communicate with his mother. Reflecting this back to young people and parents is an important step in enabling families to develop safer and more effective ways of communicating their distress, particularly where aggression has become a central tool in how families communicate.

There are a number of approaches that we could take in order to support James to develop alternative ways of communicating his pain or distress to his mother. First, the Yuva practitioner can help James to name what it is that he is trying to communicate. This might involve doing a sequence analysis of a recent occasion where James shouted at his mum, working on an 'iceberg' to explore the hidden

---

Yuva practitioner: Can you remember a time when someone was shouting at you?
James (young person): Yes.
Yuva practitioner: Can you remember what they were saying?
James: Kind of. I just remember her shouting and being really angry at me.
Yuva practitioner: So you can't remember what she was actually trying to say to you, just that she was angry and shouting – the shouting was getting in the way of the message. So when you're shouting at your Mum and you want her to hear how you're feeling, do you think she's paying attention to what you're trying to say or to the shouting?
James: I don't know, I suppose she's paying attention to me shouting but she never listens to me unless I shout, so what am I supposed to do?

thoughts and feelings that are often obscured by his anger, or by just asking James: *So if you weren't being angry at your Mum, what would you be feeling? What did you want her to understand?*

Once we have identified what James wants to communicate we can start to work on how he can deliver these messages. This involves looking at different modes of communication such as 'Aggressive', 'Passive-aggressive', 'Passive' and 'Assertive', and exploring the costs/benefits of each of these modes to present a range of choices in how to communicate. The practitioner could ask James for examples of times when he was able to communicate difficult feelings *without* shouting and explore how this worked out for him. This is likely to highlight James's communication strengths, as well as the barriers to him doing this in particular situations or particular relationships. The aim is for the Yuva practitioner to support James to come up with viable and realistic alternatives to aggression. For example, to replace shouting: *You never listen to me!* with saying: *When you talk over me I feel like you aren't listening to me.*

The key to the effectiveness of these strategies is the parents' receptiveness to their child's attempts at assertive communication. If James starts to practise healthier communication strategies with his mother and these are not positively reinforced then he is unlikely to continue using them. This will always be a challenge because many of the mothers of children who use violence and abuse will understandably struggle to be receptive to their children in times of conflict. The model of parallel work means that while James is being supported to explore communication, another member of the team can work with his mother in developing empathy and understanding of James's feelings of distress.

Exploring the function of violent and abusive behaviour

During this work it is very important to distinguish between (i) communication that intends to describe a feeling or concern and (ii) communication that is intended to make someone do something. If James's definition of 'effective' communication is that which results in him getting to do what he wants (e.g. to get money, to be allowed to go out) then he is unlikely to use alternative strategies of communication that do not result in him getting what he wants.

Therefore, an important part of our work with young people and parents is to enable them to identify the function of their abusive behaviour. With young people this can be explored through asking questions such as: *What did you get out of behaving that way? Did you get what you wanted? Did she hear you? Was she scared?* Asking such questions can help elicit young people's motivations for using abusive behaviour and explore what they gain from behaving in this way:

'When I hit her, it makes me feel better' (Jay, 14-year-old male)

'When I get angry and physically big myself up, my Dad backs off and moves away from me' (David, 15-year-old male)

TABLE 7.2 Techniques used with young people and parents to address abusive/violent behaviour

Technique	Aim and description of the technique
Ecograms	The client is asked to draw a map of their family relationships, close friends and other support networks. Using straight lines to denote family ties and squiggly lines to denote conflict, the aim is to look at what social and family networks are available. This can help to build resilience through use of 'positive' networks and reduce reliance on those members of the network who collude with, or reinforce, those beliefs that enable the young person to justify their use of violence and abuse.
Abusive Behaviour Inventory	Based on an adult domestic violence tool used at DVIP, the inventory is a document that lists 40 violent and abusive behaviours such as swearing, kicking, demanding money and strangling that young people might use towards their parents and other family members. The inventory is used with young people and parents to identify the frequency and types of abusive behaviour used by the young person (i) in the last 4 weeks and (ii) overall.
Sequence analysis of a recent violent or abusive incident	This a common technique used in cognitive-behaviour therapy. It involves a step-by-step breakdown of a recent conflict situation in terms of those feelings, thoughts and actions that are assumed to precede every behavior. Through the use of probing questions, the client describes their feelings, thoughts and actions during a particular recent incident that led to violence and abuse. The description is usually pictorially represented to show the spatial surroundings of the conflict. Probing questions might include: *Which room were you in? Where was Mum standing? What did he say? What did you say? Did you say that before or after you moved over to her side of the table? Who was standing in the doorway? Could Mum leave the room? What were you feeling just before you ran up the stairs?*
Motivational questioning	This is a counselling technique that aims to elicit motivational statements from the client and encourage them to imagine the future and identify the steps required to bring about change. For example, a young person who has not been allowed to go back home after a violent incident may be asked to imagine where he would like to be living in six months' time. This could be followed by questions such as: *What steps will you need to take before you can go back home? Can you think of a time when you were able to have a discussion with your mum without being abusive? What skills might achieve this? What new skills might you need to learn? What help and support might you need?*
Rating scales	Young people are asked to complete rating scales to identify their feelings about their current behaviours and the level of desired or actual change. For example, they might be asked to rate on a scale of 1–10: *How bad do you feel about your aggressive behaviour? How much do you want to change this behaviour? How much do you believe you can make changes to your behaviour?* Such questions distinguish between the child's intention to change and their belief in their ability to make changes.

TABLE 7.2 Continued

Technique	Aim and description of the technique
Systemic questioning	Systemic questioning is used to explore empathy and other people's perspectives. For example: *What would Mum say if she was sitting here? How would your son describe the argument you had? If she was here in this room now and I asked her how she felt when she was shouting at you, what do you think she would say?*
Deconstructing abusive language	This is used to explore the cultural attitudes and beliefs underlying abusive language. It enables parents and young people to examine attitudes to gender and sexuality that may inform patterns of power and control within their family (for example, see case study of Sofi and Jay).
Self-talk	Exploring self-talk with young people can be useful for developing a sense of agency and control over their behaviour. Examples might include asking clients to identify negative and/or destructive self-talk and helping them to identify more constructive self-talk to override this.
Watching video clips	Such techniques are useful to help visualise aggressive and controlling behaviours and identify societal influences on gender roles and how this applies to us as individuals. It is also a useful tool for exploring a young person's attitudes and beliefs about abusive behaviour when they are reluctant to talk about their own experiences.

'I know that people get scared of me when I behave like I [am a] mad person' (May, 16-year-old female)

'It keeps her in her place . . . she can't tell me what to do' (Karim, 16-year-old male)

Eliciting such statements creates a space for exploring the feelings that underpin these motivations and for considering the losses (as well as the gains) of using violence and abuse. This can also be a useful technique with parents to help them to understand the function of their child's behaviour within the family context. This involves exploring what role the child has within the family and what the outcome and consequences of their behaviour might be. Such techniques can be particularly important in families with a history of adult domestic violence where there are gendered patterns of power and control.

Conclusion: reflecting on the 'Yuva approach'

This chapter offers a reflective account of the development of the Yuva young people's service, detailing how it emerged as part of a wider programme of domestic violence support services in response to the needs of local communities and local services. The Yuva service draws on a range of theoretical and practice approaches, influenced by our location within a feminist domestic violence service and by the backgrounds of the practitioners who have helped to shape and deliver the service. We realised early in the development of the service that there was unlikely to be one model of practice that would work across all cases; a model that would work for young people in abusive intimate partner relationships, for children aged 10, 11 and 12 who are violent towards their siblings and for young adults aged 17 and 18 who are abusive towards their mothers. The complexity and diversity of our work has been difficult to capture in both detail and scope when writing this chapter, just as it presents challenges for us when training and supporting new members of staff. We hope that, in tracing the development of the service and detailing the range of techniques that we use, we have captured something of the 'Yuva approach'.

Our location within DVIP means that we have drawn on many of the resources, techniques and basic principles used in mainstream domestic violence services, such as a commitment to *parallel working* with perpetrators and victims/survivors of domestic violence and the use of particular assessment, safety planning, motivational and risk management techniques. While these resources have been integral to the development of the service, we have found the need for new conceptual models to underpin our work. The victim/perpetrator model of gendered power and control that underpins adult domestic violence work and the message that the perpetrator is always 100 per cent responsible for the violence do not usually apply in cases of child-to-parent violence. The vast majority of the young people we work with who are using violence are also victims of past or ongoing abuse, and are often struggling to manage complex and multiple support needs. The case studies of Jay and Sofi, Jane and Shanika, and Katie and her family are examples of this. However, as we have made clear, it is unhelpful to understand their violence only as a response to victimisation (Featherstone, 1997). Disentangling the categories of 'victim'/'abuser' and the constructions of 'agency'/'passivity' they give rise to is central to our work with parents and young people and to our own professional reflective practice.

As feminist domestic violence survivor practitioners and as youth workers committed to using youth-/women-centred models of participatory practice, CPV work can be extremely challenging, as it unsettles what we mean by 'woman-centred' or 'child-centred' practice. In both group supervision and as colleagues engaged in parallel work, we wrestle with how to balance women's and children's voices and rights and how to understand the role that gender plays in shaping the norms, values and attitudes that underpin the patterns of abusive behaviour that we witness. Unable to fall back on established models of practice, we continue to engage with these questions, working with each other and with clients to unpick the complex relationship between gender, power and responsibility in families experiencing child-to-parent violence.

Notes

1   At the time of writing we are funded to work in six local authority areas in London, but regularly receive referrals and enquiries from practitioners working in other authorities.

Often referrers are unable to secure funding to proceed with the referral suggesting that if funding was not restricted we would have a much higher referral intake.

2 This proportion is slightly below the average for London, which is 44.9 per cent.

3 All names have been changed to protect client confidentiality.

4 The Common Assessment Framework (CAF) is a statutory tool used by practitioners to identify a child's support needs and enable different agencies to work together to meet any identified needs.

References

DVIP. (2013). *Domestic Violence Intervention Project: Increasing the safety of women, children and young people affected by domestic abuse for 21 years: 1992–2013.* www.dvip.org [Accessed 5 September 2014].

Featherstone, B. (1997). What has gender got to do with it? Exploring physically abusive behaviour towards children. *British Journal of Social Work, 27,* 419–433.

Holt, A. (2013). *Adolescent-to-Parent Abuse: Current Understandings in Research, Policy and Practice.* Bristol: Policy Press.

Holt, A., and Retford, S. (2013). Practitioner accounts of responding to parent abuse – a case study in ad hoc delivery, perverse outcomes and a policy silence. *Child & Family Social Work, 18*(3), 365–374.

Munday, A. (2009). *Break4Change: Does a holistic intervention effect change in the level of abuse perpetrated by young people towards their parents/carers?* Unpublished BA (Hons) Professional Studies in Learning and Development dissertation. University of Sussex, Brighton, UK.

8

THE YOUTH OFFENDER DIVERSION ALTERNATIVE (YODA)

A community-based project for youth-to-family violence in Texas

Kristin Whitehill Bolton, Peter Lehmann and Catheleen Jordan

This chapter describes the development of a university–court partnership aimed at developing and testing a social service intervention called the Youth Offender Diversion Alternative (YODA). The partnership is based on participatory research principles, and it strives to include a contextual understanding of the organization, service providers and recipients. Thus, it is distinct from traditional "top-down" approaches in its goal of creating an equalitarian dynamic between the research and community partners. The core aim of the YODA program is to eliminate youth-to-family abuse and enable future desistance from crime. This chapter begins by conceptualizing youth-to-parent/family violence and identifying the key approach behind the challenges experienced in setting up the intervention, including sustainability, participant recruitment, measurement and data collection, funding, barriers produced in the negotiation of such partnerships, and attempts to expand the program to other sites. This chapter concludes by discussing factors related to program success, including prior collaboration history, court/judge buy-in, regularly scheduled communication events and data updates.

Conceptualizing youth-to-parent violence

Literature examining youth aggression as it relates to family violence primarily focuses on *youth-to-parent violence*. Youth-to-parent violence consists of behaviors that include bullying, slapping, punching, hitting, assault (which may be sexual) and causing emotional as well as physical harm (Cottrell, 2001). Young people who exhibit aggressive and/or violent behaviors may compromise their developmental growth and are at risk of continuing offending behaviors. The data on youth

TABLE 8.1 Summary of individual and systemic factors contributing to adolescent aggression

	Individual and systemic factors	Research evidence
Individual	Low tolerance for frustration	Baron & Byrne (1998)
	Lack of empathy	Evans & Warren-Sohlberg (1998)
	Escalation of anti-social behaviors	Ellickson & McGuigan (2000)
	Substance use	Pagani et al. (2004); Wei, Loeber, & White (2004)
Family	Poor family interactions	Pagani et al. (2004)
	Lack of affection and parental support	Barrera & Li (1996); Demaray & Malecki (2002)
	Authoritarian parenting	Beyers & Goossens (1999); Pagani et al. (2004)
	Intimate partner violence	O'Leary, Slep, & O'Leary (2007)
	Violence against mothers	Ulman & Straus (2003)
	Abuse of siblings	Harbin & Madden (1979)
	Overly permissive/inconsistent parenting	Cottrell & Monk (2004)
	History of parent-to-child aggression	Appel & Holden (1998); Boxer, Gullan, & Mahoney (2009); Gershoff (2002)

violence is broad, yet the statistics on prevalence suggest it is a serious health issue requiring an urgent social response (see Introduction, this volume).

There is consensus within the criminal justice and research communities that no single individual or family characteristic can predict youth aggression or youth-to-parent family violence (Unnever, Cullen, & Agnew, 2006; Chung & Steinberg, 2006). Instead, a number of factors are found to contribute towards aggressive behaviors, and these factors should be seen as interrelated as the young person proceeds through adolescence. Youth-to-parent/family violence is *systemic* and is often mediated by a number of issues. Thus, a movement towards *diversion* to address the complexity of needs in the adolescent offending population is the least intrusive and most sustainable form of intervention (Holman & Ziedenberg, 2006). Table 8.1 lists those family and individual factors that have been empirically investigated and demonstrated to be predictors of youth-to-family violence. Regarding these factors, the YODA program works to address (i) frustration, (ii) lack of empathy, (iii) anti-social behaviors, (iv) abuse of siblings, and (v) poor family interactions, depending on the results of an individualized assessment.

The Youth Offender Diversion Alternative (YODA)

Tarrant County in Texas, United States, is a diverse metropolitan area that encompasses the city of Fort Worth and other surrounding suburban areas. According to the United States Census Bureau (United States Census Bureau, 2014), Tarrant

County has a population of approximately 1.9 million and a median household income of $56,859. The racial demographic includes 76 percent White, 16 percent African American, 1 percent Asian, 5 percent Hawaiian/Pacific Islander, 28 percent Hispanic or Latino and 2 percent people of mixed race heritage (United States Census Bureau, 2014). Historically, Texas has a reputation of being "tough on crime" and, in terms of family violence, the *Texas Code of Criminal Procedure* states that "The primary duties of a peace officer who investigates a family violence allegation or who responds to a disturbance call that may involve family violence are to protect any potential victim of family violence, enforce the law of this state, enforce a protective order from another jurisdiction as provided by Chapter 88, Family Code, and make lawful arrests of violators" (1999). Police officers are required to arrest individuals if there is probable cause to believe that a violent offense has occurred, even if the family members and/or victims indicate that a violent act did not take place.

In September 2010, there were approximately 120 cases pending of young offenders charged with domestic violence of non-intimate partner family members in Tarrant County, Texas. Youth offenders charged with *misdemeanor family violence* through Tarrant County Criminal Court #5 received deferred adjudication and were typically assigned to anger management courses. Prior to the development of YODA, there were no systems of care to assess the particular short-term or long-term strengths, risks or sufficiency needs of the young offender. Likewise, there was no evidence of family involvement to explore how family functioning might help promote positive behaviors (e.g., good family ties, supportive relationships) which research suggests is a critical requirement for ending youth violence (e.g., Guerra, Kim, & Boxer, 2008). This need to better understand the factors that contribute to this growing problem led to the development of a program which aimed to promote the cessation of youth violence toward family members and to enable young people's transitions into healthy independent adulthood.

The development of a court–university partnership

In an effort to address an increase in the number of young people charged with assault against a non-intimate family member, the University of Texas at Arlington and Tarrant County Criminal Court #5 engaged in a court–university partnership, known as YODA (Jordan *et al.*, 2013). The concept of this partnership drew from *community-based participatory research* (CBPR), a collaborative approach that emerged out of public health practice. CBPR deviates from traditional "top-down" approaches in which evidence-based practice intervention strategies are developed and evaluated by researchers without strong community input or participation. The National Institute of Health (2009) defines CBPR as scientific enquiry whereby

> [C]ommunity members, persons affected by the health condition, disability or issue under study, or other key stakeholders involved in the community's

health have the opportunity to be full participants in each phase of the work (from conception – design – conduct – analysis – interpretation – conclusions – communication of results).

CBPR strives to incorporate and empower community stakeholders through equal partnerships with university researchers in an effort to collectively improve community outcomes and it includes three core components: (i) reciprocal transfer of information, including insights and expertise, (ii) joint decision-making, (iii) equal ownership of the outcomes and products of the collaboration (Viswanathan *et al.*, 2004). While offenders themselves were not part of this partnership, these core components of the CBPR model were used to underpin the court–university partnership.

The partnership was established by researchers from the University of Texas at Arlington (UTA) approaching the presiding judge of Tarrant County Criminal Court #5 (Judge Jamie Cummings) and enquiring whether there was an area of need that could be addressed (it is important to note that one of the researchers had previously worked with the Judge on a diversion program for adult male violent offenders). Judge Cummings indicated the existence of a new trend of youth violence that included misdemeanor charges of family violence toward non-intimate partner family members. A proposal was developed by a team including Judge Cummings, Deb Bezner (Program Coordinator for Criminal Court #5), Peter Lehmann (university researcher), and Catheleen Jordan (university researcher) and funding was granted by the UTA's *Innovative Community and Academic Partnerships* (iCAP)[1] fund, which sought to support pilot projects to test the feasibility of innovative interventions with hopes of eventual sustainability.

The YODA planning committee was organized and included court personnel, university researchers, graduate research assistants, and mental health professionals. The monies from the grant funded graduate research assistants, faculty time, the mental health provider's salary, and other non-personnel associated costs (i.e., assessment instruments and travel costs). Each member of the planning committee was tasked with a mutually agreed role and was involved in the development of the project timeline. The planning committee was responsible for the research process, developing and implementing the program, and maintaining communication with all relevant stakeholders. Although each committee member had a different role, each member worked toward addressing the identified area of need: *the increasing number of youth charged with misdemeanor assault against a non-intimate family member*. Clarity around the committee's mutual goal helped to enable a strong understanding of one another and a respect for each particular area of expertise.

Program overview

The Youth Offender Diversion Alternative (YODA) was launched in the spring of 2011. Each week, the designated social work provider would attend court and young offenders were given the option of (i) enrolling in YODA, (ii) proceeding to trial, or (iii) entering a one-size-fits-all anger management group for violent offenders. In contrast to the anger management group, which lasts for 8 weeks, enrollment in YODA typically lasts for 4–6 months. However, an incentive to participate was that successful completion of the YODA program would offer the opportunity to have the assault charge expunged from record, which is beneficial to the young person given the limitations that an assault charge can have on future employment. Enrollment in the program was a condition of the offender's bail bond (the sum of which varies significantly and is established by the judge). Violation of the YODA program policies (i.e., failed drug tests, re-arrest, missed appointments) would violate the conditions of the youth offender's bond and potentially lead to their removal from the program.

The young people who qualified for the program were those who had been charged with *misdemeanor family violence* and were aged between 17 and 24 years. While the Texas Penal Code (2013) states the age of criminal responsibility as 15 years, the presiding judge made the executive decision to determine an older age range for the program based on (i) the number of individuals that fell into this age range that appeared in her court and (ii) the appropriateness of the treatment model for this age group. The program was delivered in three phases:

Phase One: referral

Phase One included the referral from Tarrant County Criminal Court #5 to YODA. Prior to appearing before the judge, the young person's eligibility for YODA was determined. Eligibility was based on a number of factors including prior violent offenses, age (i.e., 17–24 years), attitude and willingness toward change, and level of competency. Each of these factors was based on the judge and district attorney's individual assessment of the young person, although there were no formal measures or instruments used to reach these conclusions. If the youth offender was deemed eligible for YODA and selected the option to participate, he/she was oriented to the program's rules and policies and given an exhaustive assessment that examined a range of issues including aggression, mental health, resilience, substance abuse, and knowledge of community resources. Assessments were administered prior to enrollment and upon completion of the program and served as a measurement of the short-term program outcomes (long-term outcomes were measured by recidivism rates). We list the assessment instruments that were used:

- **Youth Re-Unification Matrix**: This assesses the client's *basic needs* and any *risk factors* associated with his/her current living situation. Each *basic need* and *risk factor* is rated on a scale from 1 to 5 (1 = individual in crisis; 5 = individual is empowered). Domains include housing, access to food, pregnancy, school, school conflict, legal, physical health, sexual health, mental health, engagement services, life skills, substance abuse, peer conflict, family conflict, safety in the home, transportation, community involvement, stress management, decision-making, communication style, and literacy skills.

- **The Solution Building Inventory** (Smock, McCollum, & Stevenson, 2010): This assesses the client's *solution-building abilities*. The questionnaire lists 14 items that are rated on a 5-point scale from *strongly agrees* to *strongly disagrees*.
- **The Child and Youth Resilience Measure (CYRM-28)** (Resilience Research Centre, 2009): This assesses *psychosocial resources* related to individual, relational and contextual qualities. There are 28 items that are rated on a 5-point scale from *not at all* to *a lot*.
- **Multidimensional Adolescent Assessment Scale (MAAS)** (Mathiesen *et al.*, 2002): This contains 16 subscales that assess a range of areas: 1) depression, 2) self-esteem, 3) mother problems, 4) father problems, 5) suicide, 6) guilt, 7) confused thinking, 8) disturbing thoughts, 9) memory loss, 10) alcohol abuse, 11) drug abuse, 12) personal stress, 13) friend problems, 14) school problems, 15) aggression, 16) family problems. There are 177 items that are rated on a 7-point scale from *none of the time* to *all of the time*.
- **The Trait Hope Scale** (Snyder *et al.*, 1991): This measures *dispositional hope* or the belief that good things as opposed to bad things will happen. There are 12 items that are rated on an 8-point scale from *definitely false* to *definitely true*.
- **The Novaco Anger Scale and Provocation Inventory (NAS-PI)** (Novaco, 2003): This is an 85-item two-part questionnaire. The first part assesses how an individual experiences anger through measuring cognition, arousal, behavior and anger regulation. Responses are scored on a 3-point scale from *never true* to *always true*. The second part assesses the specific situations that lead to anger (disrespectful treatment, unfairness, frustration, annoying traits in others, and irritations). Responses are scored on a 4-point scale from *not at all angry* to *very angry*.

Phase Two: case management and individual therapy

Phase Two of the program involved individual case management (which included making referrals to other agencies) and one-to-one solution-focused brief therapy (SFBT) with the young person. This phase of treatment lasted from 4 to 6 months. Participants and case workers generally met once a week during the course of treatment, with case management and SFBT administered in tandem. The section on treatment (below) provides a detailed description of how SFBT was used in this context.

Phase Three: family therapy

Phase Three of the program was optional and involved SFBT family therapy. While some young people chose to participate in weekly or bi-weekly family therapy sessions in addition to individual therapy sessions, others received only individual therapy sessions. The decision to engage in family therapy was a joint decision made by the young person and his/her family, and this element was not a requirement to complete the program. In some cases, the relationship between the young person and his/her family was so fractured that there was no communication between the young person and their family: in such instances, the family often refused to participate.

Treatment model: a strengths-based approach

Strengths-based approaches attempt to "mobilize talents, knowledge, capacities, resources in the service of achieving their (the client's) goals and visions" (Saleeby, 2006: 1). Grounded in the helping profession's changing paradigm of focusing on how people achieve health and wellbeing, strengths-based approaches place a strong emphasis on finding what is *right*, *effective*, and *strong* within individuals. Solution-focused brief therapy (SFBT) evolved out of this approach and was developed by Steve de Shazer (1940–2005), Insoo Kim Berg (1934–2007), and their colleagues in the late 1970s in Milwaukee, Wisconsin (e.g., Berg, 1994; Berg & Steiner, 2003; Berg & Dolan, 2001; de Shazer, 1985, 1988). SFBT is future-focused and goal-directed, emphasizing potential solutions to the problems that bring clients to therapy. An SFBT approach assumes that all clients have some knowledge of what would make their life better, even though they may need some help (which, at times, may be considerable) to describe the details of a better life. It is underpinned by the assumption that everyone who seeks help already possesses at least the minimal skills necessary to create solutions. Therapy comprises "specialized conversations" between client and therapist and while these conversations can be about any of the problems the client brings, the focal point is concerned with developing and achieving the client's vision of a better future.

The tenets and tasks of solution-focused brief therapy (SFBT)

SFBT operates within a competency and resource-based model. It minimizes past failings and problems, and instead focuses on a client's strengths and (previous and future) successes. The focus is on working from the client's understanding of her/his concern and what the client wishes to be different (Ratner, George, & Iveson, 2012). As it relates to YODA, the following basic tenets inform SFBT practice:

- All young people are motivated toward something and all have something constructive to offer. It is the therapist's job to uncover this and, as such, it is not helpful to view young people's behaviors as *resistant*
- The focus on "change" should be concerned with the young person's desired future and their goal to be non-violent (as opposed to concern with past problems and/or current conflicts)
- Young people should be encouraged to increase the frequency of behaviors that are helpful
- No problem behavior happens *all of the time*. There are always exceptions – that is, times when the young person could have become violent but did not. These exceptions can be used by the young person and his/her therapist to co-construct solutions

- Therapists should help young people to find alternatives to current undesired patterns of behavior, cognitions, and interactions that are already within the young person's repertoire
- Small and positive changes in young people will lead to bigger and longstanding changes
- The problem of youth violence does not necessarily reflect an underlying pathology.

Given the tenets outlined above, three tasks are fundamental to engaging a young person in the process of becoming non-violent: 1) setting goals, 2) developing a preferred future, 3) identifying and building on current strengths. These tasks are reflected in the *questioning process*, which starts early on in the therapy and is a continual part of solution-building. Questions include:

1. What are your best hopes? What do you hope to achieve from being involved in the YODA program?
2. If YODA is helpful to you, what will be different? What will you have achieved?
3. What is already in place in your life, or what is already going on, that might contribute to what you want?

Using SFBT techniques with YODA: a questioning approach

As described earlier, the YODA program comprises case management, individual solution-focused brief therapy and, in some cases, family solution-focused brief therapy. Treatment is provided by a master's-level social worker (MSW) who is trained in the use of SFBT and who works with the young person throughout each step of the process. It is vital that a collaborative stance is taken throughout the intervention, and this involves having respect for what the young person brings to the process and operating a professional partnership. It is critical for the therapist to "lead from behind": knowing and having the confidence that every young person has many ideas about what needs to happen for things to change. Collaboration sets the stage for the *expectation of change*: that is, that the young person will make progress and that the outcome will be good (Ratner, George, & Iveson, 2012).

All of the techniques used throughout the YODA intervention involve *a questioning approach* (SFBTA, 2013). The deliberate and constructive use of questions forms an important part of any practitioner's toolkit and is intended to help the young person think about the changes he/she is making – in the present and in the future (Bannink, 2006). In this context, many categories of question may be applicable and should not be limited to questions that involve strengths, coping, the future, relationships, and competencies. A number of questioning techniques can help to clarify solutions and the means of achieving them. These include (but are not limited to) looking for previous solutions and exceptions, self-directed goal-setting, the Miracle and Best Hopes Question, compliments, scaling and coping questions, inviting the client to do more of what works, setting homework assignments, and offering feedback. These questioning techniques are described below:

- **Identifying previous solutions** – Regardless of the situation and event(s) that have brought the young person to YODA, there will be past stories (from another time and place) where young people have solved problems without violence in a way that made a difference. It is important to identify these stories and use them to generate future strategies.
- **Looking for exceptions** – There will also have been occasions when young people could have behaved aggressively toward a family member but did not. Thus, *something else happened* instead of the violent behavior and it is critical to capture what exactly that was.
- **Self-directed goal-setting** – It will be easier for young people to change when the goal is self-directed (as opposed to being told what to do by someone else). All YODA participants have the capacity to do something different to resolve conflicts. Thus, self-directed goals shift attention away from what cannot be done to what can be done (Lee, Uken, & Sebold, 2014). Here, each young person is asked to identify a doable goal for themselves that will improve their life, be different, and which might be noticed by others. In this context, each young person is given an opportunity to describe cognitions, behaviors or interactions from different parts of her/his life that can be used to identify new goals.
- **The Miracle/Best Hopes Question** – A staple of SFBT is the Miracle Question (MQ): *"Suppose, when you were sleeping, a miracle happened: What would you notice? What would be different?"* The MQ is intended to obtain a description of life without the problem (de Shazer, 1988). Young people are also given the opportunity to answer *"What are your best hopes from being involved with YODA?"* The Best Hopes Question (Ratner, George, & Iveson, 2012) is an extension of the MQ and also has the potential for a positive outcome.
- **The ready use of compliments** – Compliments are an important ingredient in establishing an alliance between YODA participant and therapist, and they are useful in highlighting specific hopes, accomplishments, and goals.
- **Scaling questions** – Scaling questions can help young people to judge their current situation along a continuum. The aim is to help young people to assess how things may or may not be changing and to enable them to demonstrate accountability for themselves. For example: *"On a scale of 0 to 10 where 10 means I'm totally confident I can manage my anger and 0 is it is totally unlikely to happen, where are you now?"* Scaling questions also provide an opportunity for young people to hear themselves (and not the therapist) explain, plan, and speculate on what will be the next step up for them in the process.

- *So, what's better since we last met?* – Young people are asked at the beginning of each session a variation of this question. The question is based on the assumption that any change (e.g., demonstrating non-violent behaviors) is an opportunity for the young person to talk about their improvement. It also offers an opportunity to hear if things are the same or worse – in which case, coping questions (e.g., "*How are you managing in spite of it?*") or more solution-building questions (e.g., "*What have you done to keep things from being worse?*") may be used.

- **Homework tasks and experiments** – A positive value is placed on a young person's change through the use of homework assignments. Often, young people may perform an action, watch for new behaviors, or keep track of new thoughts or ideas that might bring about change. The key is *simplicity*: homework assignments should be doable, realistic, and/or fit with a young person's goals for change (Bannink, 2006).

- **End-of-session feedback** – End-of-session feedback has two aims: first, to acknowledge the young person's qualities and achievements and, second, for the young person (and, if applicable, their family) to provide the therapist with information that will be helpful for ongoing work. Thus, questions such as "*What questions do you have for me? What have we talked about that has been helpful? Is there anything I missed today that could help?*" will help to enable that vital *expectation of change* within the young person.

Key challenges

During the course of the development and implementation of the YODA program, the planning committee encountered several challenges. The first challenge concerned participant recruitment and prior to implementation of the program it was agreed by the judge to incentivize participation by allowing YODA participants to have the assault charge removed from their record one year from completion of the program. This may well have contributed to high enrollment levels and relatively high completion levels: findings from the program evaluation conducted after 30 months revealed an overall completion rate of 67 percent. All participants who enrolled in the YODA program enrolled under the agreement that they would be involved in a research study and they signed an informed consent form. The University of Texas at Arlington's Institutional Review Board approved the study.

A second key challenge concerned measurement and data collection. The original research design included a comparison group (TAU, treatment-as-usual). However, the court staff – who administered the TAU program – were very resistant to including a data collection component to this group. This resistance stemmed from the already-overburdened employees and the limited amount of time they were able to spend with the offenders during the 8-week anger management groups. Therefore, the research design was altered and a pre-test/post-test design was employed. However, while the university researchers were charged with measuring short-term outcomes, they did not have access to the relevant judicial date to measure recidivism rates over time, which is a limitation of the evaluation.

A final key challenge concerned funding and sustainability. The original funding cycle for the evaluation program began in March 2011 and ended in May 2012. This left a 3-month period before the fiscal budget for the court would be determined by the county commissioners. Fortunately, the funder agreed to provide bridge monies to continue the program for the remainder of the court's fiscal year – otherwise there would have been disruption to treatment services and a lapse in the enrollment cycle because of an inability to pay for the social worker and corresponding supervision.

Lessons learned

A number of elements have made the YODA program a success. First, the university researchers and the court had an established relationship prior to submitting the funding grant for the YODA program. This relationship served as a foundation of trust that was beneficial in the development and implementation of a new program. Second, the key stakeholders of the YODA program established a mutually agreed-upon goal early on in the partnership. This goal was to collectively address the issue of the increase in the number of young people charged with assault against a non-intimate family member. Finally, each collaborator had a mutually agreed-upon role, with each role drawing on a specific area of expertise that was necessary for the project to be successful. The university researchers brought knowledge related to the program evaluation and the treatment model. The program evaluation was used as a resource to determine the success of the program and whether it should continue beyond the original funding cycle. The university researchers' treatment expertise enabled them to design the SFBT intervention and train the MSW therapist. The court personnel were experts in the judicial process, and the judge, the court staff, and the district attorneys worked together to develop the judicial process for the diversion program and establish it within the Tarrant County court system. No area of expertise was deemed more important or superior to another and the equal exchange of information and communication made working together successful.

Conclusion

The success of the YODA program and the university–court partnership illustrate how social problems can be addressed within communities. The most recent program evaluation was completed 30 months after program implementation and analyses of the program assessment scores demonstrated statistically significant differences between the pre-test and post-test scores on each of the aforementioned measures (see p. 139), excluding the *youth re-unification matrix* which was not used as an outcome measure. These findings were consistent with the previous 3 program evaluations which also found statistical significance. Following a review of the program evaluation, the County Commissioners agreed to incorporate the YODA MSW position in the annual Tarrant County fiscal budget for the next 2 years, which has significantly contributed to the sustainability of the program.

The researchers have attempted to expand the YODA model to other locations beyond Tarrant County, but such attempts have been limited by lack of funding. However, a new opportunity is currently being explored with the county juvenile department, where staff are interested in implementing a YODA program with a younger population, ages 10–17 years. The university researchers are currently exploring literature on younger perpetrators of family violence and considering what program modifications would be required and how YODA might best be implemented in this setting. Issues such as home vs. office visits, and treatment under the auspices of the juvenile department vs. the university, are under consideration. In sum, the researchers hope to continue to develop and refine the YODA program and assess its effectiveness against traditional treatments, which have exhibited little success. In its initial debut, YODA has shown promise in bettering the lives of youth and their families.

Note

1   See www.uta.edu/ssw/research/icap/index.php

References

Appel, A. E., & Holden, G. W. (1998).The co-occurrence of spouse and child physical abuse: A review and appraisal. *Journal of Family Psychology*, 12, 578–599.

Bannink, F. (2006). *1001 Solution-focused questions*. New York: Norton.

Baron, R. M. & Byrne, D. E. (1998).*Social psychology*. Upper Saddle River, NJ: Prentice Hall.

Barrera, M. J. & Li, S. A. (1996). The relation of family support to adolescents' psychological distress and behavior problems. In G. R. Pierce & I. G. Sarason (eds.) *Handbook of social support and the family* (pp. 313–343). New York: Plenum Press.

Berg, I. K. (1994). *Family-based services: A solution-focused approach*. New York: W.W. Norton.

Berg, I. K., & Dolan, Y. (2001). *Tales of solutions: A collection of hope-inspiring stories*. New York: Norton.

Berg, I. K., & Steiner, T. (2003). *Children's solution work*. New York: Norton.

Beyers, W., & Goossens, L. (1999). Emotional autonomy, psychosocial adjustment and parenting: Interactions, moderating, and mediating effects. *Journal of Adolescence*, 22, 753–769

Boxer, P. Gullan, R. L., & Mahoney, A. (2009). Adolescents' physical aggression toward parents in a clinic-referred sample. *Journal of Clinical Child & Adolescent Psychology*, 38, 106–116.

Chung, H. L., & Steinberg, L. (2006). Relations between neighborhood factors, parenting behaviors, peer deviance, and delinquency among serious juvenile offenders. *Developmental Psychology*, 42, 319–331.

Cottrell, B. (2001) *Parent abuse: The abuse of parents by their teenage children*. The Family Violence Prevention Unit, Health Canada.

Cottrell, B., & Monk, P. (2004). Adolescent-to-parent abuse: A qualitative overview of common themes. *Journal of Family Issues*, 25, 1072–1095.

Demaray, M. P., & Malecki, C. K. (2002). The relationship between perceived social support and maladjustment for students at risk. *Psychology in the Schools*, 39, 305–316.

de Shazer, S. (1985). *Keys to solutions in brief therapy*. New York: Norton.

de Shazer, S. (1988). *Clues: Investigating solutions in brief therapy*. New York: Norton.

Ellickson, P. L., & McGuigan, K. (2000).Early predictors of adolescent violence. *American Journal of Public Health*, 90, 566–572.

Evans, D., & Warren-Sohlberg, L. (1998). A pattern analysis of adolescent abusive behaviour towards parents. *Journal of Adolescent Research*, 3, 210–216.

Gershoff, E. T. (2002). Parental corporal punishment and associated child behaviors and experiences: A meta-analytic and theoretical review. *Psychological Bulletin*, 128, 539–579.

Guerra, N. G., Kim, T. E., & Boxer, P. (2008). What works: Best practices with juvenile offenders. In R. D. Hoge, N. G. Guerra, & P. Boxer (eds.) *Treating the juvenile offender*. (pp. 79–102). New York: Guilford.

Harbin, H. T., & Madden, D. J. (1979). Battered parents: A new syndrome. *American Journal of Psychiatry*, 136, 1288–1291.

Holman, B., & Ziedenberg, J. (2006). *The Dangers of Detention: The Impact of Incarcerating Youth in Detention and Other Secure Facilities*. JPI Report. www.justicepolicy.org/content-hmID=1811&smID=1582&ssmID=32.htm

Mathiesen, S. G., Cash, S. J., & Hudson, W. W. (2002). The Multidimensional Adolescent Assessment Scale: A validation study. *Research on Social Work Practice*, 12(9), 9–28.

Jordan, C., Lehmann, P.,Whitehill, K., Huynh, L., Chigbu, K., Cummings, J., & Bezner, D. (2013). Youthful Offender Diversion Alternative: YODA. *Best Practices in Social Work*, 9(1): 20–30.

Lee Yee, M., Uken, A., & Sebold, J. (2014). Self-determined goals and treatment of domestic violence offenders: What if we leave it up to them? *Partner Abuse*, 5, 239–258.

National Institute of Health. (2009). *Recovery Act Limited Competition: NCMHD Community Participation in Health Disparities Intervention Research Planning Phase (R24)* [online]. Retrieved from: http://grants.nih.gov/grants/guide/rfa-files/RFA-MD-09–006.html (Accessed 25 November 2014)

Novaco, R. W. (2003). *The Novaco Anger Scale and Provocation Inventory*. Los Angeles, CA: Western Psychological Services.

O'Leary, K. D., Slep, A. M., & O'Leary, S. G. (2007). Multivariate models of men's and women's partner aggression. *Journal of Consulting and Clinical Psychology*, 75, 752–764.

Pagani, L. S., Tremblay, R. E., Nagin, D., Zoccolillo, M., Vitaro F., & McDuff, P. (2004). Risk factor models for adolescent verbal and physical aggression towards mothers. *International Journal of Behavioral Development*, 28, 528–537.

Ratner, H., George, E., & Iveson, C. (2012). *Solution focused brief therapy: 100 key points and techniques*. London: Routledge.

Resilience Research Centre. (2009). *The Child and Youth Resilience Measure-28: User manual*. Halifax, NS: Resilience Centre, Dalhousie University.

Saleeby, D. (2006). *The strengths perspective in social work practice*. 4th edn. Boston, MA: Pearson.

SFBTA. (2013). Solution focused treatment manual for working with individuals. Retrieved from www.sfbta.org/research.html

Smock, S. A., McCollum, E. E., & Stevenson, M. L. (2010). The development of the Solution Building Inventory. *Journal of Marital and Family Therapy*, 36, 499–510.

Snyder, C. R., Harris, C., Anderson, J. R., Holleran, S. A., Irving, L. M., Sigmon, S. T., & Harney, P. (1991). The will and the ways: Development and validation of an individual-differences measure of hope. *Journal of Personality and Social Psychology*, 60(4), 570–585.

Texas Code of Criminal Procedure. (1999). *Family Violence Prevention.* Title 1, chpt. 5. Retrieved from: www.statutes.legis.state.tx.us/SOTWDocs/CR/htm/CR.5.htm

Texas Penal Code. (2013). Age affecting criminal responsibility. Retrieved from: www. statutes.legis.state.tx.us/Docs/PE/htm/PE.8.htm

Ulman, A., & Straus, M. A. (2003). Violence by children against mothers in relation to violence between parents and corporal punishment by parents. *Journal of Comparative Family Studies,* 34, 41–60.

United States Census Bureau. (2014). *Tarrant, Texas* [Data file]. Retrieved from: http://quickfacts.census.gov/qfd/states/48/48439.html

Unnever, J. D., Cullen, F. T., & Agnew, R. (2006). Why is bad parenting criminogenic? Implications from rival theories. *Youth Violence and Juvenile Justice,* 4, 3–33.

Viswanathan, M., Ammeran, A., Eng, E., Gartlehner, G., Lohr, K. N., Griffith, D., . . . Whitener, L. (2004). Community-based participatory research: Assessing the evidence. Evidence Report/Technology Assessment No. 99 (Prepared by RTI and University of North Carolina Evidence-based Practice Center under Contract No. 290–02–0016). AHRQ, Publication 04-E022–2. Rockville, MD: Agency for Healthcare Research and Quality.

Wei, E. H., Loeber, R., & White, H. R. (2004). Teasing apart the developmental associations between alcohol and marijuana use and violence. *Journal of Contemporary Criminal Justice,* 20, 166–183.

9

GENDER AND ADOLESCENT-TO-PARENT VIOLENCE

A systematic analysis of typical and atypical cases

Kathleen Daly and Dannielle Wade

Introduction

The gender composition of adolescent-to-parent violence is so often presumed that researchers may use de-gendered terms such as *youth*, *child* and *parent* when they are referring to a son assaulting his mother. Indeed, the growing body of research on adolescent-to-parent violence shows that the most frequent dyad is *males* (sons) assaulting *females* (their mothers or stepmothers). By comparison, male parents (fathers or stepfathers)[1] are less likely to be targets of abuse: in part, this is because their children may view them as more intimidating and, in part, because adolescent-to-parent violence is more frequent in single-parent households, where adult females are more likely to be sole heads of families (Cottrell and Monk, 2004). Although girls may assault their parents for different reasons than boys, the target of their violence is more often mothers than fathers.

The gender composition of the typical dyad in adolescent-to-parent violence recapitulates that in adult partner violence; furthermore, mothers who are assaulted by their sons may also be assaulted by their partners (or ex-partners). Researchers have identified similar dynamics in both victimization contexts, including the 'tactics of control' used (Pence and Paymar, 1986), male attitudes of superiority over females and the ongoing (not 'incident-based') qualities of violence and conflict. However, as Daly and Nancarrow (2010: 10) suggest, 'theories of male violence against women alone do not tell the whole story' of adolescent-to-parent (son-to-mother) violence. This is because adolescent violence in families is recursive: male youth may offend against their mothers, but also be victimized by their fathers, stepfathers or their mothers' boyfriends. Mothers may blame their sons' violence on these other men; at the same time, their sons and significant male adults may join together in minimizing their violence toward mothers.

What, then, of the atypical dyads in adolescent-to-parent violence? Of girls assaulting their mothers or fathers, or boys assaulting their fathers? In what ways are the dynamics of these cases similar and different from the more typical dyad? This chapter compares three typical and three atypical cases to systematically assess the following: (i) familial contexts, (ii) types of violence, (iii) parents' and youths' explanations of violence, and (iv) disclosing violence to friends or family members and reporting it to legal authorities. Following this analysis, implications are drawn for police and justice responses to adolescent-to-parent violence.

Offending and victimization

Cottrell and Monk (2004) suggest that 9 to 14 per cent of parents are 'at some point physically assaulted by their adolescent children' (p. 1072). Drawing from Australian, Canadian, and British data, Howard (2011: 3) estimates 'one in ten parents are assaulted by their children'. Boys (sons) are offenders in two-thirds of cases, and adult women (mothers) are three-quarters of parent-victims. Condry and Miles's (2014) analysis of reported offences to the London Metropolitan Police finds that son-to-mother violence comprised 67 per cent of cases; son-to-father, 20 per cent; daughter-to-mother, 11 per cent; and daughter-to-father, 2 per cent. However, caution needs to be exercised because reporting patterns may themselves vary by the gender composition of the dyad (Condry and Miles, 2014: 168). In addition, Gallagher (2004) notes that clinical samples have a higher share of male offenders than sample surveys of self-reported offending. Although males predominate as offenders in both, a higher share of females in sample surveys likely stems from the inclusion of lower-level or less serious types of offending.

To frame our analysis of offending and victimization in typical and atypical cases, we turn to key themes in the literature: familial contexts, types of violence, parental and youth explanations for violence, and disclosing and reporting violence.[2]

Familial contexts

Youth (typically sons) who are violent towards their parents (typically mothers) are likely to have experienced sexual or physical abuse by their father and have witnessed partner violence towards their mother (Cottrell and Monk, 2004; Holt, 2009; Howard and Rottem, 2008). In addition, some fathers, even when separated from a boy's mother, may attempt to undermine her parenting or verbally abuse her in front of their son. In cases when sons had contact with their father, parental conflict remained strong (Howard and Rottem, 2008). Thus, adolescent-to-parent violence occurs within a broader familial context of violence and disharmony. It is often the tip of a more systemic family violence pattern, which includes partner abuse, child abuse, and parental abuse toward children which, as Downey suggests, 'may be co-occurring or occurring over time' (1997: 76). For this reason, she argues, violence in families is 'recursive' – that is, 'mutually shaping' rather than a linear or 'cause–effect relationship'.

Types of violence

Gallagher (2004, citing Campbell, 1993) suggests that violence by a youth (typically a son) toward a parent (typically a mother) can be 'instrumental' or 'expressive'. Instrumental violence is used to control another, whereas expressive violence is depicted as a youth 'letting off steam' in inappropriate and violent ways (p. 96).[3] A similar distinction is made in research on intimate partner violence. For example, Johnson (2008) distinguishes between 'intimate terrorism' and 'situational couple violence'.[4] In the former, an abuser (typically male) uses violence or other 'control tactics' (such as threats and isolation) against a partner (typically female) 'to exercise general, coercive control' (p. 26). In the latter, 'conflict between the partners leads to an argument, the argument escalates and becomes verbally aggressive, and the verbal abuse leads to violence . . . , [but the violence] is not driven by a general motive to control' (pp. 60–61). However, Routt and Anderson (2015) distinguish control used in adult partner violence and that used by youth toward their parents. They suggest that 'the [adult] abuser uses a variety of tactics to exert control over his partner's life, . . . [but] teens coerce parents to get something they want rather than to restrict their parent's freedom and independence' (pp. 26–27). With varied binaries used to describe types of violence, we chose 'controlling' and 'reactive' as the most descriptive.

For research on girls' violence toward parents, Routt and Anderson (2015: 70) say that it is 'almost exclusively against their mothers'. Cottrell and Monk (2004: 1081) suggest that daughter-to-mother violence is 'a paradoxical response, [. . .] used to create distance from the "feminine ideals" that [are] often ascribed to [girls]' (p. 1081). Specifically, girls may view 'their mothers as weak and powerless and use abusive behaviour against them . . . to distance themselves from [an] image of female vulnerability' (p. 1082). For son-to-father violence, Cottrell and Monk (2004: 1081) suggest that boys' abusive behaviour is 'influenced by the role modelling of masculine stereotypes that promote the use of power and control in relationships', offering one example of a boy who said, 'You kind of look up to your dad. If he's rough, you are too.' The authors also suggest that although it is less frequent, sons may 'use aggression against an abusive adult man in an effort to protect [his] mother'. Another reason cited, which is relevant to both girls and boys, is conflicting childrearing styles, whereby parents 'contradict each other'. In these circumstances, youth violence may reflect 'underlying problems in the parental relationship' (Cottrell and Monk, 2004: 1085).

Although violence toward a parent can be 'defensive or retaliatory' (Gallagher, 2004: 3), little is said about a potential mutuality of aggression, that is, when both parties agree that violence is 'one way to settle the score' (Daly, 1994: 130). To be clear, by mutuality of aggression, we mean that parents and adolescents may choose to escalate an argument by fighting each other. We do not mean a temporal ordering of violence in the home that begins with parental aggression toward children, which may subsequently lead to adolescent abuse of parents, dynamics that have been studied by Brezina (1999) and Margolin and Baucom (2014).

Parental and youth explanations for violence

As Holt (2013: 73) suggests, parental explanations for their child's violence toward them is a 'tricky terrain' because the 'dominant explanation in scientific and common-sense discourse' is that abusive behaviour is rooted in a person's child-hood, for example, by 'witnessing violence between parents' (see also Holt, 2011). When sons assault mothers, women may blame themselves, citing poor parenting or other personal deficits. Ex-partners may also blame the women, and women (mothers) are more likely than men (fathers) to say that professionals blame them (Howard and Rottem, 2008, citing Furlong, Young, Perlesz, McLachlan, and Reiss, 1991). Mothers may minimize their sons' abuse: they may excuse the behaviour as outside of their sons' control because of 'inherent traits' or 'learnt behaviour' (Howard and Rottem, 2008; Routt and Anderson, 2015). Specifically, mothers attributed their son's violence to their having learned such behaviour from their fathers, with some also blaming their sons' alcohol or drug use. Women's views of their sons' abilities to control (or not control) their abusive behaviour oscillated, but most thought it was 'entrenched' and 'out of control' (Howard and Rottem, 2008: 50). Stewart, Burns, and Leonard (2007) interviewed 60 Sydney women in 1996/7 and 2001, asking about their children's violence towards them (both as adolescents and adults). The main explanation offered was the 'bad influence of a father [or] stepfather' (p. 187), although some mothers believed they had contributed to the violence because they were 'too weak'. Some cited a child's personality ('always very self-centred' or has a 'short fuse') or mental illness, or simply claimed that the abuse was 'typical male behaviour' (pp. 187–188).

For young people's explanations of their own violence, less is known. However, Holt (2013) suggests that their explanations often mirror those of their parents by referring, for example, to a history of violence in the home. In Howard and Rottem's (2008) study, all the sons blamed people other than themselves for their abusive behaviour toward their mothers. Most blamed their victim-mothers, but some also blamed siblings and school officials.

Disclosing and reporting violence

Parent-victims may deny their child's abuse, hide it from family and friends, or not initiate police contact. This occurs for many reasons, among them: self-blame for the abuse or shame (Holt, 2009) and fear of it being revealed. One consequence of denial is a parent's isolation from family and friends in order to maintain the family secret (Bobic, 2004). A parent's reasons for not reporting to officials are fear of the ways an abusive child may react when learning the abuse was reported, and not wanting a child to go through a criminal justice process (Cottrell and Monk, 2004). It is noteworthy that these circumstances – isolation, denial, and fear about what will happen if the behaviour is disclosed to authorities – are similar to those that inhibit adult females from reporting male partner violence. According to Routt and Anderson (2015: 29–30), some parents will attempt to protect themselves from an abusive child by leaving the household at certain times of the day. Calling the police is often the last resort for victimized parents and contemplated only after abuse has been occurring for some time.

Six cases of violence

The data for six cases of violence were gathered in 2001 as part of the *In-Depth Study of Sexual and Family Violence* (see Daly, Bouhours, and Curtis-Fawley, 2007; Daly and Wade, 2012). The study examined youth justice conferences for sexual and family violence in the state of South Australia. Conferences have been used there since 1994 as a diversion from court for admitted offenders, aged 10 to 17 years.[5] During a 6-month period (July to December 2001), all youth justice conferences for sexual and family violence were identified; eight sexual violence and six family violence cases were completed during the time period. For each case, the police report of the incident and the youth's criminal history were obtained; in addition, interviews were carried out with the victim[6] and with the Youth Justice Coordinator (YJC), who organized and facilitated the conference. The interviews canvassed the offence dynamics, and what occurred before, during, and after the conference. Detailed cases studies were assembled from a rich set of case materials, and here we can only sketch the highlights. An earlier paper (Daly and Nancarrow, 2010) examined three typical cases of adolescent-to-parent violence, which are re-analysed here, along with three atypical cases. Appendix 1 provides more information on the family contexts in each case.

Typical cases

Case #1: Carolyn and Des

Des (16 years old) came home one afternoon drunk. He went to change his clothes, but after having trouble putting his belt on, he became aggravated and started to punch the walls. After smashing a hole in the wall, he went to the kitchen and started to yell and name-call his mother, Carolyn, before pushing her in the chest with both hands. Carolyn attempted to call the police, but Des ripped the phone from the wall. As she tried to leave the house, Des grabbed her and pushed her against the wall, yelling 'you're not leaving the house. I'll fucking kill you'. He picked up a knife from the kitchen drawer and slammed it into the breakfast bar, just missing Carolyn's hand. She ran from the house and called the police.

Case #2: Anna and Tom

Anna heard her daughter, Tina (10 years old), yelling from another room in their home. Anna rushed to see what was happening and saw Tom (14 years old) pushing Tina into the couch. Anna intervened and argued with Tom, and he struck her with a broom handle. Anna left the house with her daughter and contacted the police. The police report says she was fearful of going back to her house on her own. A few hours later Tom was arrested.

Case #3: Shelia and Mitch

Shelia arrived home from work and ordered a pizza for dinner, which she had with her son, Mitch (15 years old). When they finished, she told Mitch that she was going to take the leftovers to her boyfriend, Bevan. Mitch got 'very mad' about this and as Shelia was about to leave the house, he said, 'You're not going'. Shelia said, 'I am going', but Mitch then grabbed her around the throat and punched her in the head. He strangled her and held her against the wall. He then released her and told her, 'Get the fuck out and don't fucking come back'. Shelia fled to Bevan's house and from there rang the police.

Atypical cases

Case #4: Ruth and Sally

Sally (13 years old) and her mother Ruth were arguing about Sally making long-distance calls to her friends, who lived in New South Wales.[7] During the argument, the phone was pulled out of the wall (the police report does not say who pulled the phone, but the YJC thinks it was Sally), and Sally began to hit her mother in the head and upper body. Ruth said she was going to leave, but Sally prevented her from doing so by 'cornering her' in the room. Sally then grabbed two knives and raised them to shoulder height. She faced her mother and said, 'I could kill you if I wanted to. I could do a murder suicide'. Ruth left the house and went to the police station to report what happened. Sally was arrested for this offence and for previous property damage to Ruth's car.

Case #5: Graham and Matt

Graham, who is Matt's stepfather, came home from his job as a cleaner just after midnight. He started to argue with Matt (16 years old) about a missing $5 note and some expensive telephone calls. The argument moved throughout the house and ended in Matt's bedroom. When Graham followed Matt into his bedroom, Matt became aggressive and abusive. Graham said he attempted to restrain Matt. They began to 'wrestle' on the bed and Matt kicked him in the leg. Matt then grabbed a fillet knife and threatened twice to kill his stepfather. Matt's mother came into the room and told Matt to let go of the knife. Matt threw it into the air, and she picked it up. She then called the police.

Case #6: Scott and Dan

Scott usually drives his son Dan (15 years old) to his job at a fruit and vegetable shop with a start time of 6am. However, Scott had told Dan some days before that if he continued to misbehave (attributed by his parents to taking an anti-depressant), Scott would not drive him to work. The day before, Dan behaved in a threatening manner towards his mother and had 'pushed' her; for this reason, Scott said he would not drive him to work. Dan asked his mother for a lift to work, but she too said she would not take him. After contacting his employer, Dan became agitated that he would lose his job. This resulted in a fight between Dan and Scott in the front yard of their house. Dan approached his father and punched him in the face and head approximately 12 times. Scott put his son into a headlock to restrain him until the police arrived. When in the headlock, Dan tried to kick his father in the face, but he could not make contact. His mother called the police.

Relating the cases to key themes in the literature

How, then, do our cases relate to key themes identified in the literature? The variables tapping into each theme are listed in Table 9.1. Drawing from the case materials (the police report, interviews with the YJC, and in one case (#3), an interview with the victim), we show evidence of the presence ('yes' in Table 9.1) or absence ('no') of the variable descriptor in each of the six cases.

TABLE 9.1 Themes and variables in typical and atypical cases of adolescent-to-parent violence

Themes and variables	Typical		Atypical			
	#1 Vic: Carolyn Off: Des	#2 Vic: Anna Off: Tom	#3 Vic: Shelia Off: Mitch	#4 Vic: Ruth Off: Sally	#5 Vic: Graham Off: Matt	#6 Vic: Scott Off: Dan
(1) Familial contexts						
a) History of abuse of victim by adult	yes (inferred)	yes	yes	no	no	no
b) History of abuse of offender by adult	yes (inferred)	yes	yes	no	yes	no
c) History of abuse of victim by offender	yes	yes	yes	yes	yes	yes
d) Length of abuse by offender is > 12 months	yes	yes	yes	yes	yes	no
e) Youth's parents were separated	yes	yes	yes	yes	yes	no
f) Current conflict between youth's biological mother and father	yes	yes	yes	unknown	no (but some negativity)	no
(2) Types of violence						
a) Type of violence (this incident)	controlling	reactive (pattern of controlling)	controlling	controlling	reactive	reactive
b) Mutual physical aggression (this incident)	no	maybe	no	no	yes	no
c) Dispute between the victim and offender over the offence 'facts' (this incident)	no	yes	no	no	yes	no

continued . . . .

TABLE 9.1 Continued

Themes and variables	Typical			Atypical		
	#1 Vic: Carolyn Off: Des	#2 Vic: Anna Off: Tom	#3 Vic: Shelia Off: Mitch	#4 Vic: Ruth Off: Sally	#5 Vic: Graham Off: Matt	#6 Vic: Scott Off: Dan
(3) Parents' and youths' explanations for violence						
a) Victim blamed her/himself for violence	no	yes	yes	no	no	no
b) Victim believed violence was outside youth's control	no	yes	yes	no	no	yes
c) Youth blamed parent	no	yes	yes	yes	yes	no
d) Youth blamed another	no	yes	yes	no	no	no
e) Professional blamed victim	yes	no	no	no	yes	no
(4) Disclosing and reporting violence						
a) Other family members knew about the violence	yes	yes	yes	unknown	yes	yes
b) A friend knew about the violence	unknown	yes	yes	unknown	unknown	unknown
c) The police been called previously for the youth's behaviour	no	yes	no	no	no	yes
d) Primary reason police were called (this incident)	change youth's behaviour	change youth's behaviour	protect self and 'wake up' youth	change youth's behaviour and protect self	prevent injury and 'wake up' youth	prevent injury
e) The victim wanted to see the youth punished (according to the YJC)	no	yes	yes	no	yes	no

(5) Reoffending

	Case 1	Case 2	Case 3	Case 4	Case 5
(a) Youth committed another family violence offence after the conference, during a 3-year follow-up period, based on official police records in South Australia	yes (considerable to same victim, within 5 weeks)	yes (father and other family member within 18 months)	no	no	no
(b) Youth committed other offences (not directed to family members) after the conference, during a 3-year follow-up period, based on official police records in South Australia	no	yes (considerable offending to non-family and perhaps family members, including property damage and assaults; sentenced to serve 8 months)	yes (larceny offences within 15 months; not known if family-related)	no	yes (property damage a year later, then trespass and carrying weapon 7 months later; not known if family-related)

Familial contexts

Variables (a) and (b) show major differences in familial contexts for the typical and atypical cases: all the typical cases were associated with a *history of abuse* of both the victim and the offender by another adult (i.e., the victim's ex-partner, and in one case, also a current boyfriend).[8] Such violence was evident in just one atypical case (#5), in which the offender had been abused by his biological father (and perhaps also by his stepfather, but information for the latter was sketchy). In addition, in case #2, Anna believed that her ex-husband had been sexually abusing his daughter.

Common to both the typical and atypical cases were variables (c) and (d), which tapped into *the ongoing nature of the violence*: in all cases, there was a history of abuse of the victim by the offender, which ranged from about 4 months (case #6) to 18 months (cases #1 and #5) or many years (inferred in cases #2, #3 and #4).

For variables (e) and (f), which tap into *family instability and conflict*, in all but one case (#6) the youth's parents had separated. All four female victims (mothers) lived in sole-parent households. In one case (#5), the boy's mother had re-partnered and his stepfather (the victim) lived in the family home. In just one of six cases (#6) did the young person live with both biological parents. In all the typical cases, *ongoing conflict between the youth's biological parents* was evident. In one atypical case (#4), there was insufficient information to know about parental conflict. In another (#5), there appeared to be no current parental conflict; but the YJC said that although 'dad hadn't been around for a long time', the youth's mother spoke negatively about the father to her son. In case #6, the youth's biological parents have continued their relationship, with no evidence of conflict between them.

Types of violence

With all cases having a history of adolescent-to-parent violence, it is uncertain what inferences we may draw about the type of violence used in any particular episode. Nor do we have sufficient information on the developmental or escalating pattern of violence over time. Thus, we infer the degree of 'controlling' or 'reactive' violence based on cues from the police offence report and histories of violence in the home that the YJCs had gleaned in their conversations with participants when preparing the conference.

In three cases, we determined that *controlling violence* was used by the youth in the immediate incident (cases #1, #3 and #4). Des (case #1) was initially frustrated, but then escalated his violence and began threatening his mother to control her and to prevent her from contacting the police. Mitch (case #3) used violence (and threats) as a way to control his mother and to get his way (specifically, he did not want his mother to leave the house to see her boyfriend Bevan, a man Mitch disliked and who had assaulted him previously). Sally (case #4) used violence against her mother to gain more freedom: she felt entitled to have more phone time than her mother allowed. In addition, the YJC suspected that Sally's mother was 'a little fearful' of her daughter. Both Sally (case #4) and Des (case #1) used threats of murder (and in Sally's case, also suicide) to persuade their mothers to act in ways they wanted. Although Matt (case #5) also used threats,[9] he did so to end the fight with his stepfather, rather than to control his actions or prevent him from leaving the house (as occurred with Des and Sally). Indeed, in case #5, the YJC believed that Matt's stepfather was controlling in the home, just as he had been controlling during the conference.

We interpret the two cases of sons who assaulted their fathers as examples of *reactive violence*. Matt (case #5) acted violently towards his stepfather in response to accusations against him and to control the specific situation: to have his stepfather leave him alone and (perhaps) to stop being physically restrained and assaulted by his stepfather.[10] Dan (case #6) acted violently towards his father after contacting his employer and learning that he might lose his job. In case #2, we interpret the immediate incident as 'reactive' in that Tom blamed his behaviour on his sister: he told the YJC that she did something that made him angry.[11] He spat on and pushed his younger sister; and when his mother Anna intervened, he struck her with a broomstick.[12] At the same time, the YJC referred to Tom as a 'very manipulative' and 'very dangerous' boy. Our inference is that Tom used controlling violence against his mother on other occasions.

An awareness of different types of violence is important for conference preparation, as illustrated in case #3. The YJC did not realize until just before the conference how manipulative and controlling Mitch and his father were. The day before the conference, the pair arrived at the conference team's office and attempted to persuade the YJC to hold the conference that day without Shelia present. The YJC was disturbed by their behaviour and comments they made about Shelia, and he decided to implement a safety plan. He showed Mitch and his father the security set-up in the conference room, pointing out the duress alarm in the room and saying that a police officer would be on the scene immediately when it was activated. On the day of the conference, a sheriff was visible in the hallway of the conference venue, and the YJC arranged that Shelia and her support person would leave before the agreement was written up and finalized 'to allow them some space and [to] get away from the building' before Mitch and his father left.

All four female victims were subject to *controlling violence* (case #2 was a reactive incident in an overall pattern of controlling violence), but the two male victims were not. Sally's violence towards her mother (case #4) was used to assert her authority and get what she wanted; it did not fit Cottrell and Monk's (2004) image of a girl wishing to distance herself from her mother and 'feminine ideals'. Matt's violence towards her stepfather (case #5) arose, in part, because of an inconsistent application of house rules by his parents, an example of what Cottrell and Monk (2004) might view as conflicting parenting styles. Matt accepted what his mother told him to do, but not his stepfather. Mutuality of aggression was apparent in case #5, when Matt and his stepfather 'wrestled' in Matt's bedroom and Graham held Matt by the throat. In case #2, Tom said that he struck his mother with the broomstick only after she struck him with it (although it is unclear from the file what happened). These were the only cases in which there was a dispute by a youth and parent about what had occurred.

Parents' and youths' explanations for violence

Two mothers (cases #2 and #3) *blamed themselves* for their son's violence, and in both cases the women had been physically abused by an adult (an ex-partner, and in case #3, both an ex-partner and current boyfriend). With just one victim interviewed (Shelia in case #3), there was too little information to know with certainty whether parent-victims felt the professionals in their cases blamed them for the violence. In Shelia's interview, she said she did not feel she was blamed by anyone, although she believed she contributed to the violence. However, the YJC recalled that Shelia said that she did not feel believed by her ex-husband and that this made the conference process difficult. Specifically, according to the YJC, Shelia said words to this effect when speaking to her ex-husband at the conference: '[It's] hard to do this, and hear you talk about it as if you still don't believe that it happened.' Drawing from the police report and the YJC interview material, we find evidence that the professionals blamed the victims in two cases (#1 and #5, discussed below).

Three victims blamed factors as being outside the young person's control. Anna (case #2) thought that her son was treating her the same way her ex-husband did. She thought that she was partly to blame for her son's violence because she did not defend herself against her ex-husband's violence. Shelia (case #3), and her ex-husband believed that Mitch had a 'chemical imbalance' that contributed to his violence. The YJC had another view, saying that Mitch 'saw dad's behaviour, learnt from it, then when dad left, Mitch took over'. Scott and his wife (case #6) blamed their son's violence on his taking anti-depressant medication, noting that his behaviour began to deteriorate when he began to take it.

In four of six cases, the young people *blamed their behaviour on the victim or another person*. Tom (case #2), Mitch (case #3) and Sally (case #4) blamed their mother-victims for the violence, and Matt (case #5) blamed his stepfather-victim. Tom also blamed his sister. Mitch accepted some responsibility for the violence, but only after his mother said that she was partly to blame because she should not spend so much time with her boyfriend Bevan. Mitch and his father also blamed Bevan. According to the YJC, at times during the conference, Sally (case #4) made 'references to [her mum's] actions which she said prompted her actions'. The YJC interpreted these comments to mean that Sally believed 'her mother had some responsibility [for her offending] from the actions that she took'. Matt (case #5) blamed his stepfather for following him into his bedroom. He said that when he is at school, he is able to walk away from situations that make him angry, but at home he could not do that with his stepfather. Matt saw his stepfather as 'the adult who could have made the decision to stop it'. In the two cases in which the victim and offender disputed the offence 'facts' (cases #2 and #5), each blamed the other.

Professionals at the conference may diffuse blame. This occurred in case #5, and perhaps appropriately so, when the YJC and the police officer blamed Matt's offending on his stepfather, Graham. During the conference, the police officer commented on Graham's potentially illegal actions towards Matt, telling him it is 'inappropriate to put pressure on someone's throat, even if you did feel at risk. You could have quite easily said "no" and got up'. The YJC believed that Graham 'wouldn't buy that, [thinking] . . . "I'm in a fight, I'll finish it"'. The YJC also thought that Graham was 'dramatizing' the offence:

> I think we made it very clear about the seriousness of the event, that this was an offence which we were surprised – given the nature of the knife – that it had come to a conference . . . He was receiving all that . . . but then instead of leaving it at that, he was basically destroying his credibility by then taking any positives that had been gained and turning them against Matt, who was by this stage beginning to become the victim in our heads . . .

Some victim-blaming by the YJC occurred in case #1. When asked if he anticipated that Carolyn, the victim, would be blamed during the conference, the YJC said: 'I'm expecting there will be [by Des, her son] . . . I suspect [that] mum's fairly flat tone, fairly negative tone, inside the house could be one that causes him to spark.' He thought that Carolyn's 'dynamics might be feeding the problem'. He also agreed with the arresting officer's observation that Carolyn 'did not want to help herself . . . like a complainer rather than an activist'.

Disclosing and reporting violence

There was insufficient information to know whether any of the six parent-victims tried to hide or deny being abused by their child (or stepchild). In Table 9.1, variable (a) for this theme shows that in all but one case (#4), at least one other family member knew about the violence. In case #4, we have no information about Ruth's relationship with any family member except her daughter. For variable (b), two of the four female victims had told a friend about the violence (cases #2 and #3); however, we lack information on this variable for the other cases.

Victims may also hide or deny abuse by deciding not to take legal action. Although all six cases had a history of violence by the youth towards their parents, in just two had the police been called before to intervene (cases #2 and #6). First-time calls to the police by victims (or by other family members) occurred in four cases, two each in typical and atypical cases.

In all six cases, it was women who called the police. In the four cases of victim-mothers (cases #1, #2, #3, and #4), the victim left the house and contacted the police while they were away from their child. In the two victim-father cases (#5 and #6), the man's wife (and the offending youth's mother) called the police from the home.

The reasons for calling the police varied and were multiple. In two cases (#1 and #2), the mothers said they sought to change their sons' behaviour. Carolyn (case #1) believed her son 'needed some help from the authorities'. Anna (case #2) told the YJC 'she wanted him to change, and she wanted it to be miraculous'. In case #3, Shelia called the police to protect herself from her son's further abuse. She said, '[I wanted to] try and wake him up. I felt horrible doing it, but if I didn't do it, he probably would have carried on doing it, and I couldn't handle that.' In case #4, Ruth wanted both to change her daughter's general behaviour and 'sexual precociousness' and to protect herself. In the two cases of violence against a stepfather and father (cases #5 and #6), their wives (mothers of the youths) called the police, fearing further injury. In addition, in case #5, the YJC said that although Sue did not want to see her son 'as a criminal, they had tried everything to get this kid to listen to them. When the knife was produced, that was the final straw'.

According to the YJC, in three cases, the victim wanted to see the youth punished. Anna (case #2) wanted her son 'to know the consequences: either he'd get locked up or his dad would have him. That was the punishment she wanted'. Shelia (case #3) 'wanted the conference to punish' her son. Graham (case #5) wanted his stepson to have 'the book thrown at him'. Thus, whatever the initial reasons were for calling the police, victims' desires for justice may change as the case progresses. Change was evident in Carolyn's case (#1): although she had called the police to 'get help' for her son, in time she wanted to know more about her legal rights when her son breached the conditions of his pre-conference bond. Then, about 5 weeks after the conference, her son arrived home at midnight, drunk and verbally abusive; he threw a dish and food around the house and told Carolyn to call the police, claiming that the house would be 'totally trashed' before they arrived. He had also broken into her house at least four times, taking food and clothing.[13] Carolyn detailed these incidents in a letter to the YJC, which led to her son being breached by the police for failing to comply with the conference agreement. When a breach of the agreement is recorded, the police have discretion to refer the original charges back to court. They did so in this case, but a year later the charges were dismissed in court.

Subsequent offending

Table 9.1 shows re-offending, as recorded by the South Australian police, during a 3-year period (up to December 2004) for all six cases.[14] In two typical cases (#1 and #2), the young person committed another family violence offence: Des against his mother and Tom against his father. Tom committed other property damage and assault offences over the next few years (some of which may have been family-related, but the file is not clear); these resulted in a sentence of 8 months to serve in detention. In atypical case #4, Sally admitted to committing six larceny offences, but it is unknown if any of these were family-related. In atypical case #6, Dan had two cases finalized in the youth court in 2003: one for property damage and another for trespass and carrying a weapon, but it is unknown if any of these were family-related. Of all six youth, the pattern of offending for Tom (typical case #2) was the most developed and entrenched. For two (typical case #3 and atypical case #5), the police record showed no offending post-conference; and for three (typical case #1 and atypical cases #4 and #6), there was post-conference offending, but it ended in 2003.

Summary and implications

Our analysis of typical and atypical cases of adolescent-to-parent violence reveals similarities and differences. The cases were similar in that a particular violent episode is part of a broader and longer-term pattern: the youth had abused the parent in the past, and conflicts and violence featured in the relationship for over a year (except one case, which was shorter). In case #2, Anna described the abuse as having gone on 'always'. In all but one case, the youths' parents had separated. In all cases where information was available, other family members knew of the violence. There was too little information to say if victims hid the violence from friends. In two cases, disclosure to friends was mentioned; both were typical cases.

The cases differed in these ways. All the victims (mothers) in the typical cases, but none of those in the atypical cases (a mother, stepfather, and father) had been abused by an ex-partner.[15] Case #5 was somewhat unusual in that the Sue (the wife of the victim in the current incident) and her son had likely experienced abuse by her former husband. All the youths in the typical cases, but just one in the atypical cases (#5), had likely been abused by their fathers and witnessed violence against their mother in the home. In one typical case (#2), it was suspected that the boy's father had also sexually abused his daughter. For all the typical cases, there was current conflict between the biological parents, but this was not apparent (or not known) in the atypical cases (although there was some negativity expressed by a mother towards her ex-partner in case #5). Two victims in the typical cases (#2 and #3) blamed themselves (in part) for the violence, whereas none of those in the atypical cases did.

We found that female victims in the three typical cases and one atypical case (#4) had experienced controlling violence from their son or daughter, with two including threats of murder. None of the male victims experienced controlling violence. A recursive pattern of violence appeared more often in the typical than atypical cases, and with it, a 'recursive trap' (Daly and Nancarrow, 2010: 169), when mothers blame themselves for (or, in some cases, are immobilized by) their sons' violence. Although all six cases had a history of violence between the youth and parent, the typical cases had compounding influences of abuse by male ex-partners towards mothers and their sons.

No clear pattern of similarities or differences was evident for other variables. Mutual aggression was apparent in an atypical case (#5) and perhaps in typical case #2, although this is uncertain. For explanations of violence, parent-victims believed it was outside a youth's control in three cases (two typical and one atypical), and youths blamed the victim in four cases (two typical and two atypical cases); and in two typical cases, they also blamed others. Parent-victims (or their partners) had mixed reasons for calling the police: to help a youth, to 'wake up' a youth, to protect themselves, and to prevent further injury. A parent-victim's interest to see a youth punished was inferred by the YJC in three cases (two typical cases and an atypical one).

The implications for police and criminal justice responses to adolescent-to-parent violence are several. First, an incident of adolescent-to-parent violence may be reported to the police for the 'first time', but the offending has been occurring for a long time. Second, justice responses (whether by conference or court actions) alone cannot repair or resolve longstanding conflicts and abuse in families, which require psychological counselling and related types of support and intervention. Third, the gender dynamics in these cases are consistent: mothers are more likely to be victims of controlling violence than fathers.

When a particular episode of violence is reported to the police and is referred to a conference or to court, it must be carefully considered. Is the current incident a type of controlling violence, or is it more situational or reactive? If the latter, is the offence embedded in a pattern of controlling violence? In general, controlling violence may require a greater degree of care, concern, and preparation in legal and therapeutic responses; and it may also require a greater degree of intervention or monitoring.

However, our analysis of post-conference offending finds no clear or consistent pattern that relates to controlling or reactive violence. Of the four cases of controlling violence against mothers, two had subsequent family violence offending; one had larceny offences, but we cannot say if any were family-related; and one had no offending at all. Of the two cases of reactive violence, one case had property damage, trespass, and weapons offences, but we cannot say if any were family-related; and one had no offending at all. With just six cases, our ability to generalize is constrained. More research on a larger set of typical and atypical cases is required to understand the complex and recursive dynamics of adolescent-to-parent violence, their implications for legal and therapeutic responses, and their relationship to subsequent re-offending.

Notes

1　Throughout the chapter, 'mother' includes stepmother; and 'father', stepfather.
2　Key themes in the literature are sourced from Howard and Rottem (2008), who examine son–mother violence exclusively; and Cottrell and Monk (2004), Gallagher (2004), Holt (2013), and Routt and Anderson (2015), who sometimes distinguish among the dyads, but not always. We use the authors' language (that is, 'youth', 'child', 'parent'), but identify the dyad's gender composition whenever possible.
3　Some also refer to adolescent-to-parent violence as 'proactive' and 'reactive'. Routt and Anderson (2015: 77) suggest that youth tend to use both types of violence against their parents at different times.
4　Johnson (2008) identifies a third category, 'violent resistance' (pp. 48–59), but this category may have less relevance to adolescent-to-parent violence.

5 In a conference, the victim, an admitted offender, their supporters, and any other relevant parties meet to discuss the offence, its impact, and how to address the offending and victimization. The conference is organized and facilitated by a Youth Justice Coordinator (YJC), with a police officer present. If a young person admits to an offence and completes the agreement, no criminal conviction is recorded.

6 As part of the agreement with the South Australian Family Conference Team, the research team interviewed only those victims in cases referred to a conference on or after 1 October 2001 (see Daly *et al.*, 2007; and Daly and Wade, 2012, for research methods, interview instruments, and preliminary findings). Of the six family violence cases, we were able to interview just one victim; two declined or were not available to be interviewed, and three were referred to a conference before 1 October 2001.

7 Sally's father lives in the state of New South Wales, and she travels there to visit him and her friends. Apart from this, no other information exists on the file about the nature of the father's relationship to Sally or Ruth.

8 For case #1, this was inferred from the interview with the YJC, who said, 'I think there was mention [of past violence]' by Des's father. The YJC also said that both Carolyn and Des did not want the ex-husband to be at the conference because 'it would just get bogged down in their warfare'.

9 Graham told the police that Matt threatened to kill him twice; Matt denies this.

10 Matt attempted to walk away from his stepfather; but when his stepfather followed Matt into his bedroom, they 'wrestled' on Matt's bed. It is not clear how fearful Matt felt during the incident, but he thought his stepfather was trying to choke him.

11 It is not clear from the file what provoked Tom's ire against his sister. The police report says he spat on her because of something she said.

12 Tom said that he struck his mother after she broke his PlayStation controller and hit him with the broomstick.

13 After the conference, although Des intermittently stayed at his mother's house, he was under strict conditions not to enter the house drunk or without her permission. Based on information in the file, Des did not have a key to the house, and thus, could only enter when his mother was there. The YJC also said that Carolyn locked her bedroom door.

14 The data were a complete record of official youth (or adult) offending in South Australia, but not officially offending outside the state.

15 There was no information on the file in case #4 to know if Ruth had been abused by her former husband.

References

Bobic, N. (2004). *Adolescent violence towards parents*. Sydney: Australian Domestic and Family Violence Clearinghouse. Retrieved November 17, 2014 from www.adfvc.unsw.edu.au/pdf%20files/adolescent_violence.pdf

Brezina, T. (1999). Teenage violence toward parents as an adaptation to family strain: Evidence from a national survey of male adolescents. *Youth and Society*, 30(4), 416–444.

Campbell, A. (1993). *Out of control: Men, women and aggression*. London: HarperCollins.

Condry, R. and Miles, C. (2014). Adolescent to parent violence: Framing and mapping a hidden problem. *Criminology & Criminal Justice*, 14(3), 257–275.

Cottrell, B. and Monk, P. (2004). Adolescent-to-parent abuse: A qualitative overview of common themes. *Journal of Family Issues*, 25(8), 1072–1095.

Daly, K. (1994). *Gender, crime, and punishment*. New Haven, CT: Yale University Press.

Daly, K., Bouhours, B., and Curtis-Fawley, S. (2007, February). *South Australia Juvenile Justice and Criminal Justice (SAJJ-CJ) Research on Conferencing and Sentencing Technical Report No. 4: In-Depth Study of Sexual Assault and Family Violence Cases*. Brisbane:

Griffith University. Retrieved from www.griffith.edu.au/__data/assets/pdf_file/0016/50308/kdaly_part2_paper17.pdf

Daly, K. and Nancarrow, H. (2010). Restorative justice and youth violence toward parents. In J. Ptacek (ed.), *Restorative justice and violence against women* (pp. 150–174). New York: Oxford University Press.

Daly, K. and Wade, D. (2012). *SAJJ-CJ South Australia Juvenile Justice and Criminal Justice Research on Conferencing and Sentencing: Technical Report No. 5: In-Depth Study of Sexual Assault and Family Violence Cases, Part II.* Brisbane: Griffith University. Retrieved from www.griffith.edu.au/__data/assets/pdf_file/0009/497484/Technical-Report-5-updated-27-Feb-2013.pdf

Downey, L. (1997). Adolescent violence: A systemic and feminist perspective. *Australian and New Zealand Journal of Family Therapy*, 18(2), 70–79.

Furlong, M., Young, J., Perlesz, A., McLachlan, D., and Reiss, C. (1991). For family therapists involved in the treatment of chronic and longer-term conditions. *Dulwich Centre Newsletter*, 4, 58–68.

Gallagher, E. (2004). Parents victimised by their children. *Australian and New Zealand Journal of Family Therapy*, 25(1), 1–12.

Holt, A. (2009). Parent abuse: Some reflections on the adequacy of a youth justice response. *Internet Journal of Criminology*. Retrieved 15 December 2014 from www.internetjournalof criminology.com/holt_parent_abuse_nov_09.pdf

Holt, A. (2011). 'The terrorist in my home': Teenagers' violence towards parents – constructions of parent experiences in public online message boards. *Child and Family Social Work*, 16(4), 454–463.

Holt, A. (2013). *Adolescent-to-parent abuse: Current understandings in research, policy and practice.* Bristol: Policy Press.

Howard, J. (2011). Adolescent violence in the home – The missing link in family violence prevention and response. Retrieved 8 December 2014 from www.adfvc.unsw.edu.au/PDF%20files/Stakeholder_Paper_11.pdf

Howard, J. and Rottem, N. (2008). *It all starts at home: Male adolescent violence to mothers.* Retrieved November 17, 2014 from www.ischs.org.au/wp-content/uploads/2012/08/It_all_starts_at_home1.pdf

Johnson, M. (2008). *A typology of domestic violence: Intimate terrorism, violent resistance, and situational couple violence.* Boston, MA: Northeastern University Press.

Margolin, G. and Baucom, B. R. (2014). Adolescents' aggression to parents: Longitudinal links with parents' physical aggression. *Journal of Adolescent Health*, 55(5), 645–651.

Pence, E. and Paymar, M. (1986). *Power and control: Tactics of men who batter.* Duluth: Minnesota Program Development.

Routt, G. and Anderson, L. (2015). *Adolescent violence in the home: Restorative approaches to building healthy, respectful family relationships.* New York: Routledge.

Stewart, M., Burns, A., and Leonard, R. (2007). Dark side of the mothering role: Abuse of mothers by adolescent and adult children. *Sex Roles*, 56, 183–191.

Appendix 1: Case background

Case #1: Carolyn and Des

Carolyn is the sole parent of Des, having separated from Des's father some years ago. Des was meant to stay at his father's house on the night of the offence because Carolyn did not want him in her home. Although his father agreed to this, Des refused to go. Des's relationship with his father has 'broken down': he does not want to live at his father's house, and his father has 'younger children from a new relationship'.

Case #2: Anna and Tom

At the time of the offence, Anna and her husband had been separated for 18 months. They have been engaged in a bitter and complicated property settlement with significant assets. Anna's ex-husband is physically violent towards Tom. Anna thought that if Tom lived with his father, he would appreciate her more. Her primary concern is her daughter Tina, whom she sees as the 'real' victim. Anna believes her ex-husband has sexually abused Tina and is trying to take her away from Anna. Anna has contacted the police before about Tom's behaviour, but never wished to make a formal complaint. On this occasion, she reported the offence to the police, but again did not wish to make a formal complaint. Rather, she asked the police to escort her home. When they arrived, a family friend was there who said there was 'family friction in the household'. Tom was arrested soon after.

Case #3: Shelia and Mitch

Up until the day after the conference, Shelia spent time with her boyfriend Bevan, who was physically abusive towards her. However, during her interview she said she had separated from Bevan the day after the conference because he had hit her 'for the first time'. According to the YJC, Shelia's son Mitch 'hates Bevan . . . [When] everything goes wrong for Mitch, Bevan's behind it'. Mitch told the police that he was trying to frighten his mother into staying at home because she was always going to Bevan's house and did not spend enough time with him. At first, Shelia did not want the police to refer the case to a conference. However, she was grateful later that Mitch did not have to go to court and potentially incur a criminal conviction.

Case #4: Ruth and Sally

Ruth has been concerned about her daughter Sally's behaviour for some time, particularly her 'sexual precociousness', 'mixing with' older men, and disappearing (sometimes for a week) with men and having sex with them. During the conference, the YJC recalled that Sally told her mother to 'answer the question' when she 'would go off on a tangent', and that when Sally was asked what she wanted to do in the future, she said, not to be 'a criminal' like her mother (there is no information on the file on her mother's offending, if this occurred). Sally could be 'eloquent and prepared to engage in discussion', but according to the YJC, she tried to 'prove her place as an adult . . . as a much older person than she actually chronologically is'. Sally does not seem to respect her mother; she wants greater liberty and autonomy.

Case #5: Graham and Matt

Graham has been living with Sue and her son Matt for over 3 years, since Matt was 13. Matt's behaviour towards Graham has, in the words of the YJC, been 'outrageous' for about 18 months. Matt has a brother, 4 years younger. The YJC thinks there is 'favouritism because the younger brother does everything he's told, when he's told. He's the glowing light'. Further, the YJC believed it was 'pretty evident that there was this dynamic between Graham and Matt, which meant that they only had to look at each other or smell each other and the buttons were being pushed'. The YJC thought that Matt had a lot of expectations placed on him about how he should behave, but 'no one had actually told him what those expectations were'. When there were inconsistency in the rules and expectations, Matt would do what his mother said and tell Graham that he did not have to listen to him because he was not his father.

Case #6: Scott and Dan

Dan lives with his mother (Leah) and father (Scott, the victim). Dan was close to his grandmother (Scott's mother), but she was 'fairly well ostracized by Leah', in the words of the YJC. Leah was the foster child of Scott's mother (that is, Leah's mother-in-law is also her foster mother), although the file does not say when she became part of Scott's family. Leah and Scott had 'put [Dan's bad behaviour] down to his medication', according to the YJC. About 4 months before the offence, Dan started taking anti-depressants. His behaviour had become difficult around this time, and the incident in this case was the last in a string of offences that occurred during a 4-week period.

10

SPECIAL CONSIDERATIONS WHEN WORKING WITH ADOLESCENT FAMILY VIOLENCE

Jo Howard and Amanda Holt

This chapter will consider the many contexts of adolescent violence and abuse towards parents, drawing together themes that have been highlighted by contributors in the previous chapters. These contexts include working with intergenerational abuse and wider family violence, working with other family members, working with adoption; exploring the intersection of culture, gender, social class and learning difficulties and physical disability, and addressing other co-occurring issues (e.g. substance misuse, mental health problems and youth offending). While there has been a recent and welcome growth in research about adolescent-to-parent abuse, the factors that shape its experience have not been thoroughly investigated, leaving the sector unclear about how best to respond to the various presentations. Much of our discussion here is informed by analysis of the existing research literature and by conversations with experienced practitioners who work in this field.

Intergenerational violence and family violence

Intergenerational abuse and violence, occurring as child abuse and/or family violence, is a common theme in adolescent violence in the home (Howard, 2011). Given the strong prevalence of adult family violence as a context to adolescent-to-parent abuse, assessment should always screen for the possibility of adult family violence as this will inform ongoing work in terms of how the intervention will proceed and who will be involved. It will also ensure safety and risk are fully accounted for.

Any intervention where there is family violence – whether the instigators are adults and/or adolescents – must be predicated on the emotional and physical safety of all family members, and 'safety planning' should always be the first priority in any intervention work. Safety planning assesses risk and safety by ascertaining the types of violence used, frequency and severity of impact, access to support and capacity to support each family member's safety. When there is wider family violence, assessment that examines who is doing what to whom, and what impact this has, is a useful way to help prioritise need and generate strategies. Thus, it is important to recognise that there is no 'one size fits all' when it comes to safety plans and they should always be (a) guided by the individual(s) who is not safe and (b) tailored to their own specific needs. If adult family violence is identified then the victim(s) should be referred to other appropriate agencies (e.g. domestic violence agencies, child social services, the police) and the adolescent should be supported through their experience of living with family violence. The adolescents' own use of violence can still be discussed, but care must be taken to avoid placing them at risk through their disclosures and to prioritise their own safety as well as the safety of others. If family members are not safe to speak freely, and if a 'safe' space is not created, adolescents risk being re-traumatised and no constructive and sustainable work can take place.[1]

Where adult family violence in the home is identified and the adolescent is now safe, then *family systems* and *trauma-based approaches* may be the most appropriate therapeutic frameworks for intervention. Family systems practice recognises (i) the recursive patterns that repeat across the generations and (ii) that a change in these patterns requires change in the parent–child relationship. This includes a mutual examination of the beliefs, values and attitudes that support the use of violence. This examination includes exploring how power is enacted in all its forms across and within each family member's relationships (see Pereira, this volume). Practitioners such as Perry (1997) and Evans (this volume) highlight the long-term impact of trauma on the developing brain and how this contributes towards the use of violence. A trauma-informed practice uses assessment to inquire about the possibility of family trauma, whether caused by family violence, grief and loss, child abuse, war and other traumatic events. Family experiences of trauma can be identified through (non-judgemental) direct questioning: 'Have you experienced family violence?' or indirect questioning: 'What happens when there's an argument at home?' Such approaches can liberate family members from secrecy and open up a space to discuss the impact of trauma.

Practitioners can explore intergenerational patterns of abuse and violence by asking the parent about their own experience of being parented: how family conflicts were resolved, how gender and power were enacted in family life, and what beliefs, attitudes and values influenced family life. Such questions can highlight that violence can be learned and that intergenerational patterns can be changed. In cases where parents have since separated, such work should also give space to the adolescent to talk about how they feel about the parent not residing in the family home – particularly if, as is likely, there is ongoing conflict in the parental relationship. Both parents need to understand that their adolescent will have a different experience and different feelings about them than they have about each other.

Psychoeducation can inform family members about the nature of trauma, its effects on the developing brain and attachment bonds, how the experience of family violence is traumatic, and how family violence negatively impacts on the mother–child relationship (Buchanan, 2008). *Psychoeducation* can also highlight how family violence can impact on a woman's ability to parent in the way she wants and can contextualise the violence: this can enable parents and adolescents to not feel blamed by others or to blame themselves. An adolescent who doesn't understand why he/she 'loses it' so easily can then make sense of their behaviours and gain hope that change is possible. At the same time, *psychoeducation* should emphasise that experience of trauma is not an excuse for the violence: adolescents must still be held accountable through a 'both/and' approach, whereby the practitioner does not get drawn into dichotomies about people's status (e.g. 'good parent'/'bad parent'; 'victim'/'perpetrator') and instead appreciates the multiplicity of understandings concerning the problematic situation. This is highly sensitive work that requires an ongoing safety lens and key focus on the emotional experience and needs of the child.

Working with other family members

As is evident from the research, parent abuse not only impacts parents, but other family members – living within or outside the family home. They may be affected through direct victimisation, or indirectly through the trauma and stress of living in a violent household. Siblings are frequently victimised (Cottrell, 2004; Howard and Rottem, 2008; Routt and Anderson, 2015) and research has documented adolescent violence towards grandparents (Gadd *et al.*, 2012) and other family members such as aunts, uncles and cousins (Jackson, 2003; Holt, 2013; Purcell *et al.*, 2014). One consequence of this is that family members may withdraw from the parent and/or young person, further isolating the parent and hampering their development of a support network (see Omer, this volume). Indeed, family members might also add to the distress itself, by colluding with the child or blaming the parent for the abuse (Howard and Rottem, 2008).

If work with parents and young people is under-resourced, then work with other family members is even more so. Support workers have expressed concerns that child protection agencies – which are statutorily responsible in cases where siblings meet the threshold of significant harm (or risk of harm) in the home – do not work in partnership with the practitioner who is responding to parent abuse because they are simply too overwhelmed with other, 'more urgent' cases of child abuse and neglect. Child protection agencies highlight the dilemma of acting in the best interests of *the child being abused* while also acting in the interests of *the abusing child*. This may result in removal of the non-offending child from the family home if the parent is unable to guarantee their safety. This short-term solution does nothing to stop the violence and further penalises parents who are themselves unsafe, as well as the children also being abused.

The importance of engaging *all* family members inside the home, and supportive ones outside the home, cannot be underestimated, given how violence affects all family members. Family members' response to the violence – to the instigator(s) and to the victim(s) of the violence – will, inadvertently or otherwise, condone or censure those behaviours. Family patterns frequently endure over generations and challenging or changing these patterns may hold a key to cessation of violence.

In a practice setting, family work may include exploring how conflict and power are enacted, how family alliances manifest, and how family beliefs and attitudes about gender, conflict resolution and styles of parenting shape the practice of violent and abusive behaviour. Family members can play a supportive role – for example, by challenging a child's abusive behaviour (see Omer, this volume), by acting as a confidante (Edenborough et al., 2008) or by offering temporary respite by housing the child (Jackson, 2003; Edenborough et al., 2008; Holt, 2013; Haw, 2010). Family members can also play a role in keeping siblings safe, promoting a united front against the violence, promoting non-violent attitudes and behaviours and by simply being 'present' in the home, rather than withdrawing and leaving other family members to cope alone.

Working with adoption

Parent abuse in the context of adoption has received little research attention. However, it is clearly of significance: a recent report commissioned by the UK Department for Education found that the most common reason for adoption breakdowns is adolescent violence towards their adoptive parents. The study, which constituted the UK's first national study on adoption breakdown, found that 71 per cent of boys and 44 per cent of girls exhibited a pattern of violent behaviour towards their adoptive parents that was 'intended to control and dominate [where] parents found they had to change their own behaviours in response' (Selwyn et al., 2014: 148).

The adoptive context means that the abuse may take particular forms and shape particular parental responses. For example, a young person may threaten parents by suggesting that a younger sibling, particularly a birth child, will be removed from the family home if the parent seeks help for the violence (indeed, Selwyn et al. (2014) document cases of siblings having to be removed from the family home because of the violence instigated by an adopted child). Parents often adopt more than one child and it is important to recognise that these children may be particularly vulnerable to an adolescent's violence – for example, if they have special needs and/or traumatic histories. Indeed, the high level of violence experienced by adoptive parents gives weight to the argument that childhood trauma is a significant determinant of adolescent-to-parent abuse.

Selwyn et al.'s (2014) study found that a significant minority of parents face false allegations made by their adoptive children in the context of parent abuse, and this devastates them, with many feeling that their ability to parent effectively has been compromised by their child's violence. Having 'passed' a whole host of 'suitability' assessments prior to the adoption, parents may feel particularly reluctant to disclose the abuse and seek support. Reluctance to seek help may be compounded by a pressure to be grateful, to be an 'extra-good' parent, and to be responsible to 'make it all OK' – something which is often reinforced by social workers and adoption support agencies. Parents may have had particularly optimistic expectations about having a child, and may be in shock at what has happened to their idealised goal of adoption. They may also feel resentful about having to *fight fires they didn't start* (Calissendorff, 2015). Parents have reported that, when they did seek help from support services, professionals minimised the seriousness of the violence and treated it as 'normal' because of the child's history. Parents have reported loss of trust and a sense of betrayal by professionals who promised so much in encouraging the parent to adopt and who offered so little support in helping the parent to manage their child's violence (Selwyn *et al.*, 2014).

Intervention work with adoptive families may present particular challenges for practitioners, who need to be aware of assumptions of biological relatedness in their work, and of other forms of sameness (e.g. ethnicity). For example, much intervention work uses exercises where parents discuss and reflect on their child's (or their own) early experiences and this is a challenge when parents do not know their child's family history (or perhaps their own). It is also likely that trauma is much more prevalent in such populations: the most common reason for entry into care is abuse and/or neglect, including exposure to domestic violence. Attachment disorders[2] are more common, though arguably over-diagnosed, in adopted children (Woolgar and Scott, 2013). Therefore, such families are particularly likely to need intervention work which recognises the impact of trauma and which focuses on developing attachment bonds (see Evans, this volume), although it may be that children and young people are not yet in a place to engage with therapy. Intervention work also needs to recognise that the development of identity in adolescence is likely to be more complex for adopted children.

Gender

The use of violence is gendered, yet part of the problem in ascertaining gendered patterns to this form of family violence lies in the definition, or lack thereof, of adolescent violence in the home, where the identity positions of 'parent' and 'child' are foregrounded and where the identity positions of 'mother' and 'son' (and so on) remain hidden. Therefore, intervention work which raises the gendered nature of adolescent-to-parent violence, particularly in relation to the main cohort being male violence against female family members, is beneficial because it supports mothers to understand that their experiences take place within a broader societal context. This should lessen the stigma and sense of failure experienced by the mother. It also offers an opportunity to discuss gendered beliefs and attitudes that influence family dynamics and relationships so that mothers and adolescents can more clearly identify some of the determinants of the violence and constraints to change.

How mothers understand their adolescents' use of violence may be shaped by their own gendered beliefs (for example, a mother may understand the use of violence as a 'male response' to stress or pressure). In practice this means that work with mothers needs to examine how they construct gender and how it has influenced the mother–child relationship and their ability to stop the violence and/or seek help. It involves an examination of the role of guilt, shame and fear of blame – for example, women who have left violent partners frequently report shame that they have 'failed' to make the relationship work and have denied their son a father (an emotional vulnerability which their child might manipulate during an abusive encounter). The beliefs and attitudes held by mothers are frequently barriers to them taking action and for this reason they need to be examined and challenged (albeit in a non-blaming context) in order to support effective change.

In a practice setting, questions that explore the notion of gendered attitudes, beliefs and behaviours in adolescent-to-parent violence may include:

- What ideas do you have about how boys should be parented by a mother?
- Do you think there's any connection between Susie abusing you and her seeing your husband constantly criticising you?
- What role does parental guilt play in maintaining violence?

Adolescents can be asked:

- What ideas about how males should deal with conflict support the violence? If other ideas took hold, would this help to stop the violence?
- Where did you get the idea that a mother should take orders from her son?
- What might be different if the relationship between you and your mum was based on trust and respect rather than on power and control?[3]

One important practice issue concerns whether – and to what extent – intervention work should be gendered, in terms of practitioners and participants. While the gender of the practitioner does not seem to have any particular bearing on successful outcomes in intervention work, group programmes usually have a male and female facilitator. This provides young people with an opportunity to model the characteristics inherent in positive gendered relationships – respect, open communication, power sharing and equality – which they may not have observed in their own family. When both facilitators cooperate and negotiate, participants can see an alternative model for gendered relationships. Having both male and female adolescents together also gives an opportunity to compare and contrast gendered views and for young people to hear and explore different perspectives. Alternatively, some group programmes[4] only work with one gender to enable more gender-sensitive resources and activities to be used to explore gender issues in greater depth and to ensure that participants feel safe where, for example, there may be a history of past abuse by the other gender (a similar argument has been made for the practice of same-sex parent programmes). More generally, it has been suggested that mixed gender participants may distract each other or block full participation, and that male and female adolescents have different ways of engaging in group programmes in terms of maturity, articulacy and degree of self-reflection. However, at present there is no evidence to suggest that same-gender groups have better or worse outcomes than mixed gender groups.

Working with cultural difference

There has been little research into experiences of parent abuse in families of minority status, but one interesting example is Ryan and Wilson's (2010) research with Māori mothers in New Zealand on which Murphy-Richards reflected (this volume). The interview approach incorporated Māori values and practices, such as beginning the interview with *karakia* (prayer) and using an interview schedule which was informed by *Te Whare Tapa Wha*: the four walls of the house.[5] Findings illustrated how perceptions of *whānau* – the extended family support which is part of Māori culture – served to exacerbate feelings of isolation and shame in mothers experiencing parent abuse. Additional pressure to maintain their *whānau* impacted on all four dimensions of their wellbeing, and attempts to seek help from outside agencies were met with institutional and interpersonal racism. Eventually each of the mothers was able to heal by sharing their stories with each other, reclaiming their *tino rangatiratanga* (self-determination) and reconnecting with their indigenous roots. Although small in scale, such research indicates how cultural contexts shape the formation and meaning of family life, including family/parental responsibilities. This in turn shapes the ways in which abuse towards parents might find its form and how families seek and respond to outside support – particularly from agencies which parents may be reluctant to contact owing to fear of cultural stereotyping and a mistrust of support workers from the majority culture (who may have a history of working in culturally insensitive ways).

Working in culturally competent ways requires practitioners to reflect on how their own cultural identity shapes their therapeutic style, techniques and emotional triggers (Hardy and Laszloffy, 1995). Of course, a practitioner's own cultural identity may be so normalised as to be almost invisible, but it is vital that practitioners reflect on how their own systemic privilege may engender particular power relations in their daily interactions with clients (Berg, 2014). Programmes for intervention developed for majority cultures may not be appropriate for families from minority cultures, and it is important to recognise that concepts such as 'empowerment' may be perceived as very *disempowering* for people in a non-Westernised cultural context. For example, Chrichton-Hill (2001) analysed the relevance of the Duluth Model and, in particular, the Power and Equality Wheels which are central to the model (see Routt and Anderson, this volume) for Samoan families living in New Zealand. She found that the four 'domestic violence' facilitators identified by the Duluth Model, such as 'objectification of women' and 'belief in natural order'[6] were less applicable to the organisation and practice of Samoan family life. This can result in intervention programmes that do not reflect Samoan experiences or build on the existing strengths of Samoan women (Chrichton-Hill, 2001).

We know from domestic violence research that participants in support programmes who are from minority communities may not be familiar with particular terminology, and may interpret the same words differently[7] (Kasturirangan *et al.*, 2004). Participants may not speak the dominant language and this may limit their engagement in group programmes (as well as their engagement with printed materials). In such circumstances, translators may be used, but it is important that professional translators (rather than family members) are used to support open and safe conversations.[8] The impact of significant change, such as migration, or the experience of war and persecution can lead to social isolation or poverty, both of which enable adolescent-to-parent abuse. Families may be fearful of authorities, may have lived in countries that do not have supportive services, may feel it is inappropriate to seek help from strangers and/or may fear reprisals from government, services or from their own communities. Such fears may be particularly profound if coupled with concerns over undocumented immigration status.

Social class, socio-economic status and poverty

The role of social class and socio-economic status (SES) in parent abuse has not yet been widely explored in the literature, particularly where it interacts with variables such as culture, gender or 'race'. While some practitioners have commented that their clients are more middle-class than they would expect (see Gallagher, this volume), it is likely that social class mediates the kind of support and resources that parents seek out. The role of social class and help-seeking has been more clearly articulated in adult family violence research, with findings suggesting that women with access to more resources have more options available to them, and this includes the option of defining the behaviour or particular situations as unacceptable or intolerable (in contrast, families living in poverty with few resources may have less freedom to define the situation as intolerable since there is little possibility of the problem being solved) (Liang *et al.*, 2005). However, it is important to recognise that the relationship between SES and help-seeking is a complex one, and families who are relatively privileged may face particular challenges: for example, middle-class families may experience greater self-blame and humiliation because they feel domestic abuse *shouldn't* happen to families who are privileged (Weitzman, 2000). Furthermore, while families with greater material resources have opportunities to seek help from private therapists, such options nevertheless serve to privatise family violence, which can (further) isolate the victim and maintain the status quo of family violence as an individual and silenced struggle (Berg, 2014).

In terms of practice, practitioners should be mindful of the ways that financial hardship might impact on families' ability to engage. Families may require casework in order to support them with financial difficulties, they may require transport to appointments and they may be unable to afford to take time off from jobs or afford childcare during intervention sessions. Some programmes, such as Do it Different (Wakefield, UK) and Keeping Families Safe (Melbourne, Australia), offer food as an incentive for young people's engagement, and have found that this strategy has a positive impact on attrition rates of young participants.[9]

The intervention work itself might also acknowledge participants' own socio-economic context and its relationship to family outcomes: for example, we know that neighbourhood socio-economic disadvantage can be have a negative impact on parenting (including style, monitoring and supervision), on physical and psychological health and on the forging of social connections (Edwards and Bromfield, 2010). All of these factors may exacerbate family stress and conflict, hamper families' ability to engage in intervention work, and help enable adolescent-to-parent abuse to continue, and as such it might be worth exploring with family members in a supportive setting.

Working with learning difficulties and physical disabilities

Parenting a child with a disability presents its own challenges, and parents must navigate a whole host of educational, health, social and personal challenges that are unimaginable to other parents. Both the joys and the strains of parenting may be more pronounced when parenting a child with a disability, and when the stress of parenting a child with a disability is compounded by other stresses, psychological distress is a potential outcome for both mothers and fathers (Singer *et al.*, 2007). While in *some* cases of *some* developmental disabilities a child's aggressive behaviour may be part of their symptomatology (Brosnan and Healy, 2011), we also know that children with disabilities are far more likely to be victims of violence and abuse than children without disabilities (Jones *et al.*, 2012; Son *et al.*, 2012). Similarly, parents with disabilities are more vulnerable to violence and abuse both inside and outside the family home (Hughes *et al.*, 2012) and, of course, this may make them more vulnerable to abuse and violence from their child. Indeed, the parents of children with severe behavioural problems often view themselves as having less power than their child (Bugental and Lewis, 1998).

Parents of children with a disability often believe that the disability 'causes' the violence and that they are powerless to effect change. While disability may contribute to the use of violence, it is uncommon that behavioural modification cannot stop or reduce the use of violence. Work with disability may involve working with the parent to explore (i) their understanding of the disability and its relationship to violence and (ii) what behaviours are a component of the disability and which have been learnt and therefore can be changed. Young people can be supported to learn skills such as self-calming, improved communication and time out. In some cases medication may be an adjunct to violence cessation or an end point in extreme high-risk situations.

Whether working with parents or young people with disabilities, practitioners can face additional challenges. Where family members have physical disabilities, the physical space and any resources and materials need to be made accessible. In the case of learning disabilities, groupwork may not be appropriate and, in such cases, work on a one-to-one basis can be offered, while another family member (e.g. a grandparent) can be offered a place on the group.

Having a parent with an illness or disability can produce poor emotional outcomes for adolescents, particularly if they have little choice in their caregiving responsibilities (Ireland and Pakenham, 2010). Parent abuse in cases of parents' chronic, long-term and terminal illnesses (e.g. cancer) has been documented. Practitioners may also encounter families where the parent is caring for extended family members who have illnesses and/or disabilities, which adds to family stress and depletes parents' abilities to find resources to care for themselves. Such contexts may also impact on safety issues where, for example, a parent cannot leave the house during a violent episode because they cannot leave a sick or elderly relative in the house.

Mental health/illness and substance misuse problems

It is impossible to discuss mental health problems and substance misuse separately: it is now widely acknowledged that where substance misuse issues occur, mental health issues are almost always present, particularly anxiety and depression. This is referred to as 'dual diagnosis'. Substance misuse is both a contributor to mental health problems and a way to 'self-medicate'. Adolescent substance use may impact on adolescent violence in the home in two ways: *physiologically*, impacting on brain and behaviour, and *interpersonally*, in terms of its contribution to conflicted family relationships. Many parents have reported that substance use increases the severity of abuse (Cottrell and Monk, 2004; Haw, 2010) and that a young person's substance use instigates conflicts with their parents which, in turn, produce violent encounters (Pelletier and Coutu, 1992).

In a practice setting, an adolescent who misuses substances to a significant level may lack motivation and capacity to address their use of violence. They may be at a 'pre-contemplative' stage of change[10] and the role of the practitioner is to move them to a 'contemplative stage', where an adolescent can consider the benefits and losses that substance misuse brings, including the contribution that substance use makes to their use of violence. Co-working with an alcohol and drug support worker may help progress this and create momentum for change. Parents can be supported to address their adolescent's behaviour in a way that supports change and minimises family conflict. *Psychoeducation* can be helpful for the adolescent and parents to understand the effects of problematic substance use while also working to enhance family safety. Parents require support to be able to take a stand against the use of violence and not fall into the trap of excusing, minimizing or justifying the violence because of these other issues.

In terms of mental health, it is important that these issues are not conflated with 'aggression' (see Murphy-Edwards, this volume). Research has found that if mothers understand the parent abuse in terms of their child's mental illness, they are more likely to tolerate the abuse and respond sympathetically (Stewart *et al.*, 2007). As many contributors to this volume have commented, many children and young people who exhibit violence towards parents will have received a psychiatric diagnosis, often in early childhood. However, existing research which asked parents about their experiences of mental health support in the context of adolescent-to-parent abuse has produced worrying findings: parents have reported feeling blamed (Cottrell, 2001; Howard and Rottem, 2008), feeling misunderstood as to the nature of the situation (Haw, 2010), feeling that their child was not given a sufficiently strong message about his/her own responsibility for the abusive behaviour and its impact on the family (Edenborough *et al.*, 2008) and feeling that their child was 'pitted against the parent' because of the use of 'individual-focused' rather than 'family-focused' therapeutic approaches (Edenborough *et al.*, 2008). Parents have also expressed concern that, because their child refused to engage, the mental health worker was unwilling to continue (Haw, 2010), or that, because their child behaved 'as sweet as an angel' during assessment, no further action was taken (Holt, 2011). The conflation of mental health problems, substance use issues and adolescent violence may contribute to families being passed from agency to agency, as each agency identifies the 'problem' as not fitting within their remit. Such practices may be particularly prevalent in 'austerity contexts' where there are insufficient resources to deal with even the most straightforward of cases.

In terms of practice, both mental health and substance use problems require assessment to ascertain the capacity of the adolescent (and parent) to engage in interventions. It is important that practitioners investigate the context of the abusive behaviour and its possible conflation with other issues to understand whether the behaviours have any neurological or psychiatric foundation. An alcohol and drug assessment will ask about the types of substances used, how they are administered, the frequency of use and impact on family relationships and capacity to engage and actively participate in intervention work. Adolescents who use violence in the home may also come from families where parents have mental health and/or substance misuse issues. This impacts on capacity to parent and may increase friction in the family home. Again, where parental issues are present, intervention should address these issues and explore their relationship, if any, to the adolescent's use of violence.

Youth offending and youth justice

Research that has explored the relationship between adolescents' use of violence in the home and risk of, or actual, youth offending has not produced consistent findings. While some studies suggest that those who have been arrested for offences related to adolescent violence in the home are likely to have previous offences for violence (e.g. Kennedy *et al.*, 2010) or delinquency (e.g. Evans and Warren-Sohlberg, 1998), other studies have found that such offenders have *significantly fewer* or *no previous offences* compared to adolescents who commit other kinds of offence (e.g. Gebo, 2007). Furthermore, research from Spain suggests that young people who are involved in the justice system because of parent abuse-related offences have a *different profile* from those in the justice system due to other offences (Contreras and Cano, 2014; Ibabe *et al.*, 2014).

However, it is often during youth justice casework for other offences that practitioners first discover that the young person they are working with is violent towards his/her parents. Thus, where young people are already involved in the youth justice system, assessment should always consider the possibility of adolescent family violence. While parents and families can be a conduit to changes in offending behaviour, this is harder to enact when parents are frightened and feel powerless. Parents are frequently blamed for young people's offending, and they are frequently made accountable for their child's behaviour through the use of parental responsibility laws. In such a context of blame and 'responsibilisation' (Garland, 2001), it is unsurprising that parents feel unable to disclose the violence as an additional family issue.

Given the central role that the youth justice system has in a) identifying cases of adolescent violence in the home and b) offering family support for 'families in trouble', one important question concerns whether the criminal justice system is the most appropriate arena for the provision of support for parent abuse. While most practitioners would agree that keeping adolescents away from court-mandated interventions is best practice, where adolescents are *already involved* with youth justice services, it is important to be ready to respond to the possibility of youth violence (and this readiness includes 'asking the right questions' at the assessment phase). Interventions for adolescent-to-parent abuse should be flexible and offer a 'sliding scale' of approaches from voluntary early intervention strategies to a mandated criminal justice response for more severe and entrenched cases. An Australian study, *The Last Resort* (Howard and Abbott, 2013), showed that when a clear message is given by the criminal justice system that antisocial and violent behaviour is not acceptable and when adolescents and family members are supported to access counselling services, more positive outcomes eventuate. Programs such as Step-Up (see Routt and Anderson, this volume) illustrate the benefits of using court-mandated interventions as a diversionary measure to avoid further criminal justice involvement, but not all court-mandated intervention work is effective: studies have found that young people who have prior arrests and who truant from school are least likely to complete family violence intervention programmes (Nowakowski *et al.* and Mattern, 2014). However, court-mandated programmes certainly seem to be a more effective step than the use of court-mandated injunctions, which one recent study identified as having a high breach rate (32 per cent) and a high percentage of applications being abandoned due to reluctance by applicants (usually the victim) to proceed (Purcell *et al.*, 2014).

Notes

1 If violent adults are still living in the family home, it is important to unpick the motivation behind the adolescent's violence, as it may be born of self-defence, or the attempt to protect other family members.
2 *Reactive attachment disorder* is categorised as a *trauma- and stressor-related disorder* in DSM-5. It has two subtypes: emotionally withdrawn/inhibited (*reactive attachment disorder*) and indiscriminately social/disinhibited (*disinhibited social engagement disorder*). Both subtypes

are the result of early childhood neglect that limits a child's ability to form attachments (American Psychiatric Association, 2013).

3 Jenkins (1990) discusses such invitational questions in his book *Invitations to Responsibility*. While his approach relates to work with violent men, it is useful for working with adolescents who behave violently. Alternatively, PACT, an intervention programme in Leeds, England, uses questions derived from *The Boy Code* by William Pollack (1998) – termed 'The Lad's Law' – to explore what it is to grow up male, before asking them what they think 'The Mum's Law' might look like (Jenny Bright, pers. comm., 23 November 2014).

4 Examples include Step-Up Ballarat (Victoria, Australia) and Parents and Children Together (PACT) (Leeds, England).

5 *Te Whare Tapa Wha* incorporates four dimensions: *Taha Tinana* (physical wellbeing), *Taha Hinengaro* (mental wellbeing), *Taha Whanau* (family wellbeing) and *Taha Wairua* (spiritual wellbeing) (Ryan and Wilson, 2010).

6 The other two cultural facilitators are 'forced submission' and 'overt coercion and physical force' (see Pence, 1985: 8).

7 This issue also applies to other minority groups, where terms of class, 'race' and gender, for example, the concept of *empowerment* may have a different resonance for participants than for the practitioner.

8 An important complexity to consider in such cases is that the child may act as a language broker for the parent, and the abuse of this role may form an important part of the abusive context.

9 Do it Different also found that, by beginning each session with the young participants and the facilitators dining together around a family table, it acts as a powerful attachment symbol of a 'good family' and contributes to the sense that the group is a 'safe base' for the young men to experiment with new behaviours (Group worker, pers. comm., 10 December 2014).

10 This refers to Prochaska and Di Clemente's (1985) influential *stages of change* model that was initially developed in relation to addiction and behaviour change. The stages are (i) pre-contemplation (ii) contemplation (iii) preparation for action (iv) recent change (v) maintenance.

References

American Psychiatric Association. (2013). *Diagnostic and statistical manual of mental disorders* (5th edn.). Washington, DC: Author.

Berg, K. (2014). Cultural factors in the treatment of battered women with privilege: Domestic violence in the lives of white European-American, middle-class, heterosexual women. *Affilia: Journal of Women and Social Work*, 29(2), 142–152.

Brosnan, J. and Healy, O. (2011). A review of behavioral interventions for the treatment of aggression in individuals with developmental disabilities. *Research in Developmental Disabilities*, 32(2), 437–446.

Buchanan, F. (2008). *Mother and infant attachment theory and domestic violence: Crossing the divide*. Australian Domestic & Family Violence Clearinghouse, Australia.

Bugental, D. B. and Lewis, J. C. (1998). Interpersonal power repair in response to threats to control from dependent others. In *Personal control in action* (pp. 341–362). New York: Springer.

Calissendorff, S. (2015). *I didn't start the fire: Parenting an adopted child with reactive attachment disorder*. [Blog] Institute for Attachment and Child Development. Available from: http://instituteforattachment.org/i-didnt-start-the-fire-parenting-an-adopted-child-with-reactive-attachment-disorder/ [Accessed 6 May 2015].

Crichton-Hill, Y. (2001). Challenging ethnocentric explanations of domestic violence: Let us decide, then value our decisions – a Samoan response. *Trauma, Violence, & Abuse*, 2(3), 203–214.

Contreras, L. and Cano, C. (2014). Family profile of young offenders who abuse their parents: A comparison with general offenders and non-offenders. *Journal of Family Violence*, 1–10.

Cottrell, B. (2001). *Parent abuse: The abuse of parents by their teenage children*. Ottawa: Family Violence Prevention Unit, Health Canada.

Cottrell, B. (2004). *When teens abuse their parents*. Halifax, Nova Scotia: Fernwood.

Cottrell, B. and Monk, P. (2004). Adolescent to parent abuse. *Journal of Family Issues*, 25, 1072–1095.

Edenborough, M. D, Jackson, D., Mannix, J. and Wilkes, L. (2008). Living in the red zone: The experience of child-to-mother violence. *Child and Family Social Work*, 13, 464–473.

Edwards B. and Bromfield, L. (2010). Neighbourhood influences on young children's emotional and behavioural problems. *Family Matters*, 84, 7–19.

Evans, D. and Warren-Sohlberg, L. (1988). A pattern analysis of adolescent abusive behaviour towards parents. *Journal of Adolescent Research*, 3(2), 201–216.

Gadd, D., Corr, M. L., Fox, C., & Butler, I. (2012). *From boys to men: Phase three key findings*. Manchester: University of Manchester School of Law.

Garland, D. (2001). *The culture of control: Crime and social order in contemporary society*. Oxford: Oxford University Press.

Gebo, E. (2007). A family affair? The juvenile court and family violence cases. *Journal of Family Violence*, 22(7), 501–509.

Hardy, K. V. and Laszloffy, T. A. (1995). The cultural genogram: Key to training culturally competent family therapists. *Journal of Marital and Family Therapy*, 21(3), 227–237.

Haw, A. (2010). *Parenting over violence: Understanding and empowering mothers affected by adolescent violence in the home*. Patricia Giles Centre: Perth, Australia.

Holt, A. (2013). *Adolescent-to-parent abuse: Current understandings in research, policy and practice*. Bristol: Policy Press.

Howard, J. (2011). *Adolescent violence in the home: The missing link in family violence prevention and response*. Australian Domestic & Family Violence Clearinghouse, Australia

Howard, J. and Abbott, L. (2013). *The last resort: Pathways to justice. Adolescent violence in the home*, Peninsula Health, Victoria.

Howard, J. and Rottem, N. (2008). *It All Starts at Home: Male Adolescent Violence to Mothers*. Research report, Inner Couth Community Health Service Inc. and Child Abuse Research Australia, Monash University.

Hughes, K., Jones, L., Wood, S., and Bellis, M. A. (2012). Violence against individuals with disabilities: A synthesis of studies on prevalence and risk. *Injury Prevention*, 18 (Suppl. 1), A142–A143.

Ibabe, I., Arnoso, A., and Elgorriaga, E. (2014). Behavioral problems and depressive symptomatology as predictors of child-to-parent violence. *European Journal of Psychology Applied to Legal Context*, 6(2), 53–61.

Ireland, M. J. and Pakenham, K. I. (2010). Youth adjustment to parental illness or disability: The role of illness characteristics, caregiving, and attachment. *Psychology, Health & Medicine*, 15(6), 632–645.

Jackson, D. (2003). Broadening constructions of family violence: Mothers' perspectives of aggression from their children. *Child and Family Social Work*, 8(4), 321–329.

Jenkins, A. (1990). *Invitations to responsibility: The therapeutic engagement of men who are violent and abusive*. Dulwich Centre Publications.

Jones, L., Bellis, M. A., Wood, S., Hughes, K., McCoy, E., Eckley, L., Bates, G., Mikton, C., Shakespeare, T., and Officer, A. (2012). Prevalence and risk of violence against children with disabilities: A systematic review and meta-analysis of observational studies. *Lancet* (8 September), 380 (9845), 899–907. DOI: 10.1016/S0140–6736(12)60692–8

Kasturirangan, A., Krishnan, S., and Riger, S. (2004). The impact of culture and minority status on women's experience of domestic violence. *Trauma, Violence, & Abuse*, 5(4), 318–332.

Kennedy, T. D., Edmonds, W. A., Dann, K. T. J., and Burnett, K. F. (2010). The clinical and adaptive features of young offenders with histories of child–parent violence. *Journal of Family Violence*, 25(5), 509–520.

Liang, B., Goodman, L., Tummala-Narra, P., and Weintraub, S. (2005). A theoretical framework for understanding help-seeking processes among survivors of intimate partner violence. *American Journal of Community Psychology*, 36(1–2), 71–84.

Nowakowski, E. and Mattern, K. (2014). An exploratory study of the characteristics that prevent youth from completing a family violence diversion program. *Journal of Family Violence*, 29(2), 143–149.

Pelletier, D. and Coutu, S. (1992). Substance abuse and family violence in adolescents. *Canada's Mental Health*, 41, 6–12

Pence, E. (1985). *The justice system's response to domestic assault cases: A guide for policy development.* Duluth, MN: Minnesota Program Development.

Perry, B. (1997). Incubated in terror: Neurodevelopmental factors in the 'cycle of violence'. In J. Osofsky (ed.) *Children, youth and violence: The search for solutions.* New York: Guilford Press, pp. 124–148.

Pollack, W. S. (1999). *Real boys: Rescuing our sons from the myths of boyhood.* New York: Henry Holt & Company.

Prochaska, J. and Di Clemente, C. C. (1985). Processes and stages of change: Coping and competence in smoking behavior. In S. Shiffman and T. A. Wills (eds.) *Coping and substance use.* New York: Academic Press, pp. 319–343.

Purcell, R., Baksheev, G. N., and Mullen, P. E. (2014). A descriptive study of juvenile family violence: Data from intervention order applications in a children's court. *International Journal of Law and Psychiatry*, 37(6), 558–563.

Routt, G. and Anderson, L. (2015). *Adolescent violence in the home: Restorative approaches to building healthy, respectful family relationships.* New York: Routledge.

Ryan, R. G. and Wilson, D. (2010). Nga tukitanga mai koka ki tona ira: Māori mothers and child to mother violence. *Nursing Praxis in New Zealand*, 26, 25–35.

Selwyn, J., Wijedasa, D., and Meakings, S. (2014). *Beyond the Adoption Order: Challenges, Interventions and Adoption Disruption.* London: Department for Education Report.

Singer, G. H., Ethridge, B. L., and Aldana, S. I. (2007). Primary and secondary effects of parenting and stress management interventions for parents of children with developmental disabilities: A meta-analysis. *Mental Retardation and Developmental Disabilities Research Reviews*, 13(4), 357–369.

Son, E., Parish, S. L., and Peterson, N. A. (2012). National prevalence of peer victimization among young children with disabilities in the United States. *Children and Youth Services Review*, 34(8), 1540–1545.

Stewart, M., Burns, A., and Leonard, R. (2007), Dark side of the mothering role: Abuse of mothers by adolescent and adult children. *Sex Roles*, 56(3–4), 183–191.

Weitzman, S. (2000). *Not to people like us: Hidden abuse in upscale marriages.* New York: Basic Books.

Woolgar, M. and Scott, S. (2013). The negative consequences of over-diagnosing attachment disorders in adopted children: The importance of comprehensive formulations. *Clinical Child Psychology and Psychiatry*, doi: 10.1177/1359104513478545.

11

WORKING WITH ADOLESCENT VIOLENCE AND ABUSE TOWARDS PARENTS

Reflections and concluding thoughts

Amanda Holt

When attending conferences and workshops on this topic, I often observe passionate debates regarding how to work with adolescent violence and abuse towards parents. To what extent should we focus on the histories of family members? When should we use a group programme, and when might such work be better undertaken in a one-to-one setting? Is it most effective to work with parents, with the adolescent, or with both? Should we work with family members together or separately? At what stage in the child's development is it appropriate to *name this problem* and intervene? How much attention should we pay to issues of gender in our understanding of the problem and in the way we organise our practice? Of course, these are important debates to have, and many of them have been explored in this volume. However, sometimes such debates can obscure areas of significant agreement about what is appropriate and effective when working with this problem. It may be surprising that there is already some consensus given that practice in this field is in its infancy. However, it is clear that the specialist work discussed in this volume has been developed from our significant knowledge built over years of working in the fields of adult domestic violence, youth justice and family support. Therefore, I would like to focus my reflections on a number of areas where there does appear to be agreement across the chapters in this volume, regardless of therapeutic approach and context of intervention. I hope that what emerges from this consensus is something that starts to look like 'good practice(s)'.

The importance of safety planning, assessment and engagement of families

In any work with family violence in the home, the key priority needs to be the *safety* of all family members. Before intervention work can start, practitioners need to help family members to find ways to ensure their safety. Aside from practical measures such as developing a 'safety plan' (i.e. what family members can do/where they can go during a crisis situation), there needs to be acknowledgement that intervention work itself may be 'risky'. Sometimes it may be too risky and such work may need to be postponed (see chapter by Howard and Holt). At other times, it may involve the recognition that, particularly at the beginning of intervention work, abusive and/or violent behaviour may escalate in response. *Assessment* is integral to safety planning and, in their chapter, Whitehill Bolton, Lehmann and Jordan describe a number of assessment tools they use in their intervention programme. However, 'checklist-style' assessment tools should always be used in conjunction with (and not as a replacement for) meaningful conversations and observations that explore the context of the violence and abuse. This might include precipitating factors (such as mental health issues), family dynamics and communication styles, family histories (including violence and abuse), an awareness of the structural locations of family members (e.g. status relating to gender, dis/ability, sexuality) and any cultural issues that might require specialist input. While assessment should always include the exploration of safety issues, it is also vital for developing an intervention that is appropriate to the particular needs of family members, and this may include the application of inclusion and exclusion criteria.

Many of the contributors to this volume also highlight the importance of *family engagement* which, preferably, is voluntary. Of course, voluntariness may not always be an option and it might be appropriate for a court to sanction engagement with a programme (see chapters by Routt and Anderson and Whitehill Bolton *et al.*). However, as many of the contributors to this volume point out, intervention work is more effective when *all* family members are engaged with, or at least supportive of, the work being done. With such work, refusals are common and drop-out rates can be high. Some of this can be countered by engaging in substantial preparatory work, which may involve a number of meetings with individual family members to discuss what the intervention involves and to explore family members' concerns about participating. Potential barriers to engagement may also need to be addressed. These might include personal barriers (e.g. the cognitive function of family members, substance misuse problems); cultural barriers (e.g. language, mistrust in services); practical barriers (e.g. lack of transportation, cost, operational hours); and barriers which are unique to this problem, such as fear of perceived consequences of engagement (for example, multiple stigma, retribution by family members and unwanted intervention from statutory services).

Working in a policy vacuum

While research and practice have been developing at a steady pace over the past 20 years or so, recognition at policy level has been slow. As Murphy-Edwards describes in her chapter, policymakers across the global North are increasingly recognising the need to respond to the enormous social problems of domestic abuse and violence against women and girls (VAWG). Many governments at national and local level have developed strategies to ensure that their responses to these problems are coordinated, funded and embedded in their work. However, within this remit, attention is rarely paid to adolescent violence and abuse towards parents, and in some cases policy guidance specifically excludes those cases where it involves family members who are children. For example, the most recent UK government definition of *domestic violence and abuse* excludes those under 16 years of age (Home Office, 2013). Many of the contributors to this volume reflect on their experiences of working in a policy vacuum, something that is encountered across all national/ regional contexts and organisational settings. The lack of articulation of abusive behaviour towards parents in official discourse presents a number of challenges. These include difficulties in obtaining funding and resources to help families; problems in establishing robust prevalence data; limitations in establishing standards of practice across all intervention work; deficiencies in existing government-funded services' responses to the problem (such as schools, social services, police); and an increased sense of despair for families who seek support from their government and find little recognition of their circumstances.

Evaluation, development and supervision

Collective understanding and knowledge about abusive behaviour towards parents is still in its infancy. For that reason, there are few robust evaluation studies that can tell us about the effectiveness of different ways of working with this problem, although Weinblatt and Omer's (2008) randomised control trial for the use of NVR training is an exception (see chapter by Omer). The few evaluation studies that do exist, while incredibly useful, are difficult to interpret in light of self-selecting samples, high attrition rates, small sample sizes, lack of long-term follow-up and a lack of differentiation between different kinds of family contexts and pathways. In my previous book (Holt, 2013: 138), I examined the common factors which family members and practitioners claimed had helped instigate change, summarised as: *Naming the abuse*; *Being listened to and listening to others' experiences*; *Developing strategies to establish boundaries with young people*; *Developing self-care strategies*; and *Education about the dynamics of parent abuse*. The small-scale research studies that informed this analysis were produced by Paterson *et al.* (2002), Monk and Cottrell (2006), O'Connor (2007), Munday (2009) and Priority Research (2009) and I would advise readers to seek out these studies to find out more about how such interventions might be evaluated and what challenges are involved when undertaking such research. It is arguably even more difficult to calculate the financial 'costs and savings' when evaluating intervention work, although such estimates are essential when communicating with policymakers and grant funders. Recent research by Wilcox and Pooley (2015) estimated that €195,362 ($221,016)[1] of savings were made from running four Break4Change intervention programmes over a six-month period. This figure was broken down into €97,691 savings to children and family services, €79,305 savings to criminal justice services, €15,245 savings to health services and €3,121 to housing services. Such economic analyses usefully highlight the extent to which adolescent abuse and violence towards parents (and other family members) can impact on so many different areas of personal and social life if it continues unchecked.

One challenge for practitioners who wish to evaluate their programmes is ensuring 'programme fidelity': that is, making sure that the interventions being delivered and evaluated are standardised. However, the methodological demands of rigorous research might inhibit innovative practice. Although most of the contributors to this volume describe clear ways of working based on established therapeutic principles, they also describe an openness to trying new ideas and tailoring techniques to meet clients' needs. Particular interventions may also need to reflect local or national circumstances and many of the contributors to this volume reflect on how their own regional context shapes their practice (see chapters by Pereira, Murphy-Edwards and McGeeney, Barakat, Langeland and Williams).[2] Thus, while it is important to evaluate what works at this early stage of collective knowledge, it is important not to hamper the possibilities of experimentation and combining different approaches. For example, many concerns have been raised about the use of restorative justice in work with domestic violence because of the risks of enabling further abuse (Daly and Stubbs, 2006). However, restorative justice has been found to be successful in youth justice work, perhaps because its principles of reintegration are considered to be particularly transformative when used with adolescents, and research suggests there is potential for its use with adolescent abuse and violence towards parents (see Morris, 2002; Doran, 2007; Daly and Nancarrow, 2009). As Routt and Anderson's chapter highlights, if safeguards are put in place, there is scope for nurturing a wider 'restorative practice' framework in which to embed particular intervention strategies.

Given the complexity of the lives of families who are experiencing this problem, it may also be appropriate to use different therapeutic approaches at particular stages of development, whether in terms of individual family members' development or in terms of the family's trajectory as a whole. As some of the chapters in this volume highlight, referral for other related issues (e.g. substance misuse, bereavement, marital problems) may be necessary alongside or following intervention work. Consideration also needs to be given to how we will follow up families and provide longer-term support if necessary. Intervention work may make a difference for a while, but research does not yet tell us how families fare months or years later. If relationships deteriorate some time after intervention work has ceased, families may feel more in despair than ever. We might also begin to explore how we can develop support work in contexts other than in face-to-face settings. Few studies have explored indirect support for adolescent abuse towards parents, but there is some research evidence on the usefulness of SMS support (Howard et al., 2010), online parenting forums (Holt, 2011) and telephone support (Parentline Plus, 2010).[3] Similarly, recent work in developing online interventions for preventing abusive behaviour by adolescents also shows promise (e.g. Broeck et al., 2014; Lira et al., 2014).

While looking at developments in practice, it is worth perhaps considering whether there is a need for standards of practice. It is hoped that many of the programmes, approaches and techniques outlined in this volume will be rigorously evaluated and rolled out to meet growing demand. While this might signal progress, it is likely that such work will be undertaken by less experienced practitioners and we need to be mindful of how we can offer guidance and support to practitioners who are new to this field to ensure that this careful work is carried out with minimal risk to families. Of course, while standards of practice are one possibility, this should not replace supervision for practitioners undertaking this kind of work. Requirements for supervision vary across sectors, but as the chapter by McGeeney *et al.* highlights, supervision is particularly helpful when practitioners are grappling with a 'new' issue such as this and where answers to questions concerning norms, values, power and responsibility are still up for grabs.

The joys of working with adolescent abuse and violence towards parents

However carefully one attempts to communicate about adolescent abuse and violence towards parents, it inevitably becomes talked about in terms of *problems*: 'problem families', 'problem home lives', 'problem parenting' and so forth. Indeed, in an attempt to help it reach the status of *social problem* (and obtain the attention and resources that social problems garner), in this book I refer frequently to *the problem of* adolescent abuse and violence towards parents. Therefore, it may seem counterintuitive to claim that a common theme in this volume is the joys of such work. Yet the passion and the optimism emanating from every page are hard to avoid. I see the same passion and optimism whenever I attend conferences and workshops on this topic. As I highlight in the Introduction, many of the contributors have been working with few funds or resources to help them in the development of their unique practice. For many, their journey has been frustrating, difficult and, at times, professionally isolating. What has kept them going is their engagement in their work and their satisfaction in observing that families function better following their work with them. Indeed, their optimism is written into their practice, and the use of a strengths-based approach is advocated, implicitly or explicitly, by each of the practitioners who contributed to this volume. Approaches that focus on all of an individual's and a family's positive attributes can only be successfully utilised if the practitioner *knows* that there is more to each family than *the problem*. It's a big ask, but I hope that all of us who work in this field and who communicate with media organisations, policymakers, practitioners and researchers can develop a 'strengths-based approach' in our communication about *the problem* and those who are affected by it.

For practitioners who work in related fields and who come across adolescent abuse and violence in their caseloads, the possibility of developing their own intervention work can be daunting, particularly if they are working with little institutional support or resources. Whether working in criminal justice, child protection, victim support or in counselling and mental health settings, research suggests that professionals have varying levels of confidence in identifying abuse and violence towards parents and in developing ways to intervene effectively (Holt and Retford, 2013; Wilcox and Pooley, 2015). However, what is evident from the practitioners who contributed to this volume is that effective work can be done with little (or no) funding, resources, or even a waiting list. In his chapter, Gallagher describes how he started small – with four mothers – and developed his practice from there. There are also pockets of support all around, and the Resources section at the end of this book may be a useful first step in finding out where these are.

This book began with a Foreword by Barbara Cottrell, and I want to close the book with a quotation from her study with families experiencing teen abuse towards parents:

> You can get over a fight with your mom quicker than with anyone else. If you fight with a friend, you don't talk for a long time. Teens take their parents for granted. They take out their aggression on their parents because parents will forgive them. (15-year-old teen)
>
> (Cottrell, 2001: 12)

For me, this quotation highlights the enduring strength of the child–parent bond and suggests that there is hope: with help and support, that bond can be built on in a way that enables families to find peace with each other.

Notes

1 Calculated at a current exchange rate of 1 EUR = 1.13 USD.
2 Further examples are provided by a recent pan-European study that explored how local contexts shape the delivery of particular interventions. For example, a small Swedish community where 'everyone knows everyone' required special consideration of confidentiality and how participants share personal histories (Mortensen and Christoffersen, 2015). Similarly, in Bulgarian communities where parents had left to find work in western Europe, the caregivers who were experiencing abuse were primarily grandparents. This produced its own challenges around the adaptation of materials which were originally designed for work with parents (Assenova and Tabekova, 2015).
3 Although this particular study did not evaluate responses to parent abuse separately from other parenting support needs.

References

Assenova, A. and Tabekova, D. (2015). Raising awareness of child to parent violence in Bulgaria. Paper presented at Responding to Child to Parent Violence: European Perspectives. 28–29 January 2015. University of Brighton, UK.

Broeck, E. V. D., Poels, K., Vandebosch, H., and Royen, K. V. (2014). Online perspective-taking as an intervention tool against cyberbullying. In B. K. Wiederhold and R. Riva (eds.) *Annual review of cybertherapy and telemedicine 2014: Positive change: Connecting the virtual and the real* (pp. 113–117). Amsterdam: IOS Press.

Cottrell, B. (2001). *Parent abuse: The abuse of parents by their teenage children.* Ottawa: Family Violence Prevention Unit, Health Canada.

Daly, K. and Nancarrow, H. (2009). Restorative justice and youth violence towards parents. In J. Ptacek (ed.) *Restorative justice and violence against women* (pp. 150–176). Oxford: Oxford University Press.

Daly, K. and Stubbs, J. (2006). Feminist engagement with restorative justice. *Theoretical Criminology*, 10 (1), 9–28.

Doran, J. E. (2007). *Restorative justice and family violence: Youth-to-parent abuse*, Mount Saint Vincent University, Unpublished MA.

Holt, A. (2011). "The terrorist in my home": Teenagers' violence towards parents – constructions of parent experiences in public online message boards. *Child and Family Social Work*, 16 (4), 454–463.

Holt, A. (2013). *Adolescent-to-parent abuse: Current understandings in research, policy and practice.* Bristol: Policy Press.

Holt, A. and Retford, S. (2013). Practitioner accounts of responding to parent abuse – a case study in ad hoc delivery, perverse outcomes and a policy silence. *Child and Family Social Work*, 18 (3), 365–374.

Home Office (2013). *New Government Domestic Violence and Abuse Definition.* Home Office: London. Circular HO 003/2013. Retrieved from: www.gov.uk/government/uploads/system/uploads/attachment_data/file/142701/guide-on-definition-of-dv.pdf (6 February 2015)

Howard, J., Friend, D., Parker, T., and Streker, G. (2010). Use of SMS to support parents who experience violence from their adolescents. *Australian Journal of Primary Health*, 16 (2), 187–191.

Lira, L. R., de Iturbe, P. F., Celis, K. F., and Cortés, E. R. (2014). Evaluation of an online intervention to prevent violence in young people and adolescents. Preliminary results on its effectiveness with health professionals. *Salud Mental*, 37, 189–198.

Monk, P. and Cottrell, B. (2006). Responding to adolescent-to-parent abuse: A qualitative analysis of change factors. *Canadian Social Work*, 8 (1), 1–12.

Morris, A. (2002). Children and family violence: Restorative messages from New Zealand. In Strang, H. and Braithwaite, J. (eds.). *Restorative justice and family violence* (pp. 89–107). New York: Cambridge University Press.

Mortensen, U. and Christoffersen, I. (2015). Implementing the Break4Change programme in Sweden. Paper presented at Responding to Child to Parent Violence: European Perspectives. 28–29 January 2015. University of Brighton, UK.

Munday, A. (2009). *Break4Change: Does a holistic intervention effect change in the level of abuse perpetrated by young people towards their parents/carers?* Unpublished BA (Hons) Professional Studies in Learning and Development dissertation. Sussex, UK: University of Sussex.

O'Connor, R. (2007). *Who's in Charge? A group for parents of violent or beyond control children.* Southern Junction Community Services, Adelaide, Australia.

Parentline Plus. (2010). *When family life hurts: Family experience of aggression in children.* London: Parentline Plus.

Paterson, R., Luntz, H., Perlesz, A., and Cotton, S. (2002). Adolescent violence towards parents: Maintaining family connections when the going gets tough. *Australian and New Zealand Journal of Family Therapy*, 23, 90–100.

Priority Research. (2009). *Evaluation of SAAIF (Stopping Aggression and Antisocial Behaviour in Families).* Sheffield: Priority Research/North Essex Partnership NHS Foundation Trust. Retrieved from: www.theministryofparenting.com/wp-content/uploads/2012/02/1109-SAAIF-evaluation-Report.pdf (5 February 2015).

Weinblatt, U. and Omer, H. (2008). Nonviolent resistance: A treatment for parents of children with acute behaviour problems. *Journal of Marital and Family Therapy*, 34 (1), 75–92.

Wilcox, P. and Pooley, M. (2015). *Responding to Child to Parent Violence: Executive Summary*. Available from: www.rcpv.eu

APPENDIX

Resources

Resources from the contributors

Step-Up: a counselling programme for teens who are violent at home (US)

Includes curriculum materials and resources for practitioners, and offers training for practitioners who wish to set up their own Step-Up programme

www.kingcounty.gov/courts/step-up.aspx

Eddie Gallagher's homepage (Aus)

Offers information for practitioners on training and workshops, advice and strategies for parents (including details of support services) and research papers

www.eddiegallagher.id.au/

School of Non-Violent Resistance (Israel)

Offers details on certificated training in non-violent resistance and Haim Omer's research publications in a range of languages

www.nvrschool.com/int/

Wish for a Brighter Future (UK)

Support organisation that offers one-to-one support sessions for young people and their families. Also offers a 13-week 'parent abuse' parenting support group in collaboration with Single Person Action Network (SPAN) and Bristol City Council (Bristol).

www.wishforabrighterfuture.org.uk

Jane Evans also runs her own blog, *Parenting Post Trauma*, which offers information, audio-visual resources and training for practitioners

www.parentingposttrauma.co.uk/

Euskarri Centre for Intervention in Filio-Parental Violence (Spain)

Provides information, audio-visual material, training for practitioners and published research

www.euskarri.es/

YUVA (UK)

A domestic violence support organisation that offers one-to-one support for young people and their parents

http://dvip.org/yuva-programme.htm

Adolescent Violence in the Home (AVITH) (Aus)

Provides training for those working with AVITH, as well as information, further contacts, research reports and practical strategies for parents and young people

www.kildonan.org.au/programs-and-services/child-youth-and-family-support/family-violence/adolescent-violence/

Other resources for practitioners

Holes in the Wall (UK)

A blog run by a professional social worker that provides updates on research, practice and policymaking developments – also available on Twitter (@HelenBonnick)

http://holesinthewall.co.uk/

RecURRA Ginso (Spain)

Offers support to families who are experiencing abuse and violence from their children. Also produces research and provides resources, training for practitioners and a residential centre for young people.

www.ginso.org/

RESPECT (UK)

A membership association for domestic violence prevention programmes and integrated support services. Offers regular conferences and training for practitioners who are working with young people who use violence in close relationships (including with parents)

http://respect.uk.net/work/respect-young-peoples-service/

Responding to Child to Parent Violence (Europe)

The website for a pan-European research project that explores different ways of working with CPV across Europe. The website features research findings and reports, conference presentations, practitioner resources and training opportunities.
http://respect.uk.net/work/respect-young-peoples-service/

Sociedad Española para el Estudio de la Violencia Filio-Parental (Spanish Society for the Study of Filio-Parental Violence)

Society that aims to promote the study, teaching and research of, and ethical regulation and intervention in, filio-parental violence. Holds conferences, publishes research and provides a researcher and practitioner network
http://sevifip.org/

INDEX